TROUNCING DIABETES

The Comprehensive Practical Guide To Sustainable Conquest

Discover Life-Saving Truths You Must Know About Diabetes

Dr Festus Olubode

Appreciation

I would like to take a moment to acknowledge and thank God for the gift of life, and for being the ultimate source of inspiration for this book; **Trouncing Diabetes: The Comprehensive Practical Guide To Sustainable Conquest.** I am deeply grateful for His guidance and wisdom throughout this journey.

To my mentor, Dr Kabiru Sada, Consultant Endocrinologist, thank you for reviewing this book despite your busy schedules. Thank you for your expert guidance and recommendations- these have added immeasurable weights to the substance of this book.

I also want to thank Mrs Oluwatomilayo Desalu for her invaluable contribution to this book. Your expertise and contribution to the dietary management of diabetes in this book are greatly appreciated, and I am genuinely grateful for your insights.

Thank you, Dr Toyin Obafemi, for editing this book and for nudging me in the direction of its publication. I have held your calm and collected demeanour in admiration since our days in medical school. Thank you, and God bless you.

Temitayo, my love, I want to use this medium to thank you from the bottom of my heart, for your unwavering support, and for being a shoulder to lean on. I could not have done this without you by my side, encouraging, supporting and believing in me every step of the way. You are truly amazing, and I feel so lucky and blessed to have you as my wife. Thank you for everything, my love.

Dedication

I dedicate this book to my past and present patients and to all those living with diabetes around the world. Your unwavering determination, tenacity, and courage to confront diabetes head-on, despite the challenges and adjustments that come with it, is truly inspiring. You are the real heroes and heroines of our time. Without your strength and resilience, this book would not exist. Thank you for being an inspiration.

Table of Contents

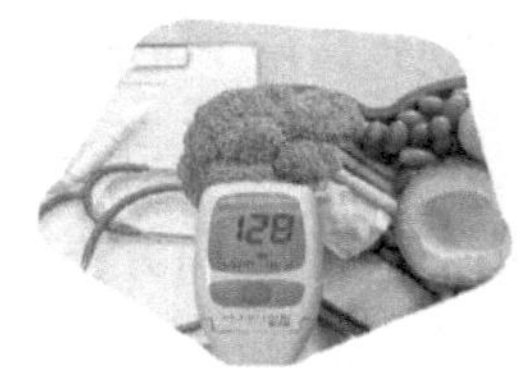

CHAPTER ONE

Historical Background

THE AIM OF THIS BOOK

"Wherever the art of medicine is loved, there is also a love for humanity."- Hippocrates

Diabetes Mellitus is one of the most extensively studied diseases in the world today. Once considered a death sentence in centuries past, a great deal of research and study over the last two centuries has brought us to where we are now. While there is still no cure, we can now safely manage the disease.

I want you to know that with the current advances in diabetes treatment, you can lead a normal life. This book is meant to empower you with the knowledge you need to add life to your years and possibly even add years to your life.

Everyone deserves to live a healthy life, regardless of their blood sugar status, and that's what I hope to give you with this book.

I want you to feel supported and informed, like a trusted friend guiding you towards better health.

It is widely believed that knowing about a disease can significantly increase a patient's confidence in managing it. For those with diabetes, being well-informed about their medical condition can help them feel more confident in facing it and following through with their treatment plans.

This, in turn, can help mitigate the risks associated with the medical condition. So if you or someone you know is living with diabetes, do not hesitate to seek the correct information - this could make a difference in managing the condition confidently.

In this book, I aim to bring both my knowledge and experience to fore. My knowledge comes from a deep understanding of the disease and the research conducted to unravel its peculiarities. My experience, on the other hand, stems from years of managing and interacting with people living with diabetes in real-life situations.

I hope that this combination of knowledge and experience will provide valuable insights into the disease and help those living with it to better manage their condition.

I do not only care about managing your diabetes; I also care about your overall health and well-being, including your physical, mental, and emotional state. Diabetes can have a negative impact on every aspect of your life, which is why this book is not just about managing the condition but also about empowering you to live your best life with diabetes.

My goal is to instill in you the confidence and grace to live with diabetes and care for yourself. You can be happy and live a fulfilling life, even with diabetes. The days when diabetes was a death sentence are long gone.

Even if you do not have diabetes, I intend to educate you about what diabetes is all about so that you may have the necessary understanding and compassion to support those around you who may be affected by it.

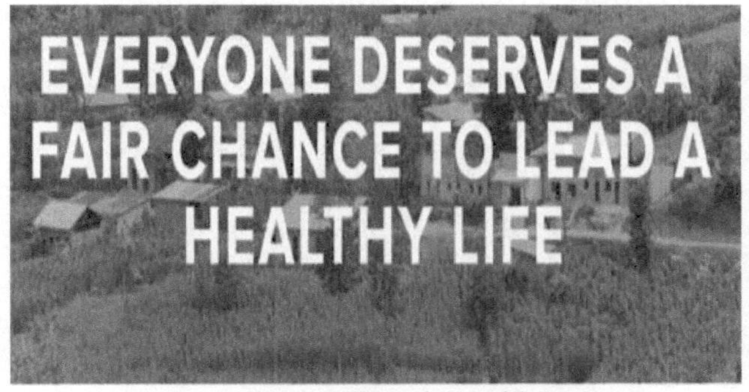

Source: Atlantic Fellows for Health Equity

HISTORICAL BACKGROUND

Diabetes Mellitus is a disease that has been known since ancient times, as descriptions were found in Egyptian, Chinese, and Indian medical texts. The name

"Diabetes" is derived from the Greek word meaning "to pass through," while "Mellitus" comes from the Latin word for "sweetness" or "honey." This is because too much glucose is found in the urine and blood of those with the condition. It was even called the "pissing evil" in the 17th century. It was also called the "wasting away" disease due to the weight loss associated with it.

In 1552 B.C., Hesy Ra, an Egyptian physician, was the first to document that frequent urination is a symptom of an unknown disease that also causes weight loss. Around the same time, other healers observed ants around the urine of individuals with this condition.

In the 2nd century, Arateus of Cappadocia (81-133A.D.) coined the term "diabetes" to describe the condition of flesh liquefying into the urine. Later, in the 17th century, Thomas Willis used the same word to describe the sweet taste of the urine of those with the disease, which was detected by water tasters. This was the major method of diagnosing diabetes at the time.

From then on, scientists began to study the disease, with some believing that it was a disease of the kidneys while some thought it was a disease of the blood. However, in 1889, Joseph v. Mering and Oskcar Minkowskwi discovered that dogs whose pancreas were removed died of diabetes. This discovery then shed light on the function of the pancreas in controlling blood glucose levels.

Then, in the 18th century, an English Doctor opined that the disease occurred in people who had injured their pancreas. In the same century, Dobson noted that diabetes is fatal in some people while it is a chronic condition in others, lending credence to the differences between Type 1 and Type 2 diabetes.

THE DISCOVERY OF INSULIN

Early treatment included exercise, if possible, on horseback as recommended by the Greek physician because they believed this would reduce frequent urination. In term of dietary management of diabetes, recommended diets were those that we now know to be inimical to the management of diabetes as the then dietary prescription comprised majorly of fat and it was noted that this was leading to severe health complications.

In 1910, Edward Albert proposed that diabetes developed when there is inadequacy of a particular chemical produced by the pancreas, and he called the chemical insulin.

Frederick Banting, a Canadian Surgeon, and Charles Best, a medical student at the University of Toronto extracted pancreatic cells from a healthy dog and introduced them into a dog with diabetes and this was found to control the diabetes. On July 27,1921 they were able to successfully isolate insulin for the first time.

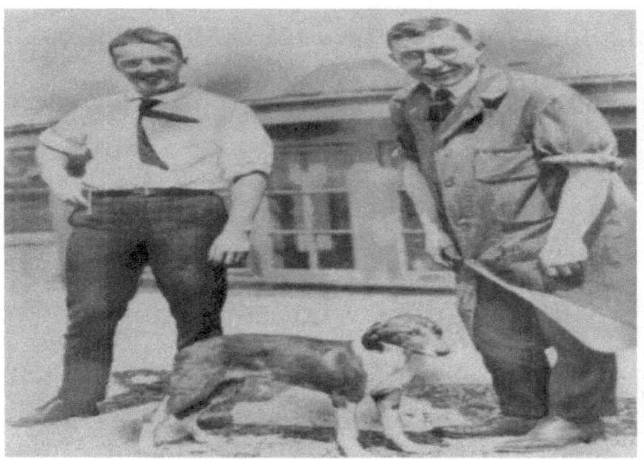

Picture showing Banting and Best. Courtesy of Toronto Star

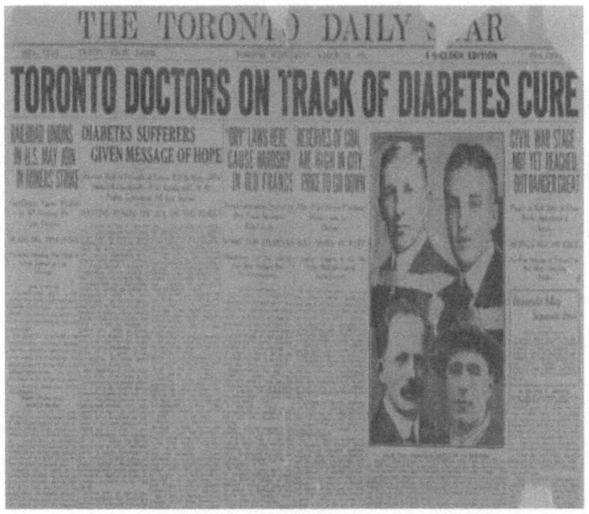

The Toronto Daily Star of March 22, 1922 Reporting The Discovery of Insulin. Courtesy of Toronto Star

By January 11,1922 Leonardo Thompson, a 14-year-old living with Type 1 diabetes became the first individual to receive insulin to treat diabetes, culminating into successful treatment of diabetes, a disease that had been deemed fatal for decades upon decades. In 1923, Banting and alongside Macleod, who was instrumental in the isolation, were awarded the Nobel Prize for Medicine or Physiology. Banting shared the award money with Charles, who as a student was not included in the award.

World Diabetes Day is celebrated annually on November 14 in honor of Sir Frederick Banting, which coincides with his birthday. This day is dedicated to raising global awareness about diabetes, emphasizing the significance of prevention, management, and research efforts

In 1923, Eli Lilly became the first Pharmaceutical company to produce Insulin in commercial quantities.

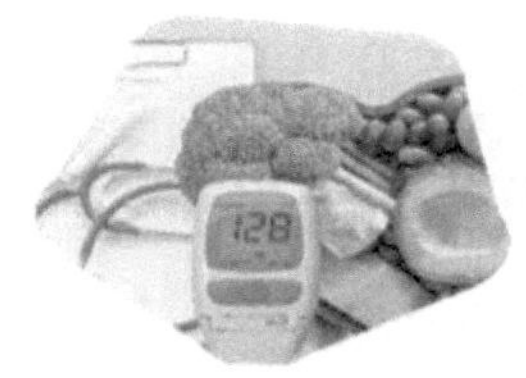

CHAPTER TWO

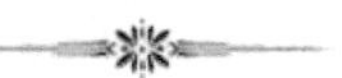

Diabetes Mellitus

DEFINITION

Diabetes Mellitus (DM) is a disorder in which the body's chemical processes are disrupted, resulting in a class of long-term diseases characterised by higher-than-normal blood sugar (glucose) levels. This disrupts the way the body processes carbohydrates, protein, and fat.

When you consume a carbohydrate-rich meal, your body digests it to produce glucose (blood sugar), which is then absorbed by your cells with the help of a chemical hormone called insulin. Insulin assists in driving the blood sugar into your body cells, thereby enhancing its assimilation.

WHAT LEADS TO DIABETES?

The Pancreas, an elongated organ situated at the back of your stomach, produces insulin. It performs mainly two functions- secretion of digestive hormones, which help with food digestion, and insulin production, which works to regulate blood sugar levels.

Blood sugar increases when the pancreas produces little or no insulin or when the body cells do not respond to insulin function. This absolute or relative insulin deficiency leads to elevated blood sugar levels called *hyperglycaemia*. Thus, Diabetes Mellitus (DM) is the persistence of hyperglycaemia.

DM can lead to medical emergencies and, in the long run, can cause damage to various organs in your body, such as the brain, eyes, heart, blood vessels, kidneys, nerves, and more.

Also, diabetes can suppress your immune system, making you vulnerable to recurrent infections. It is essential to manage diabetes effectively to reduce the risk of these complications.

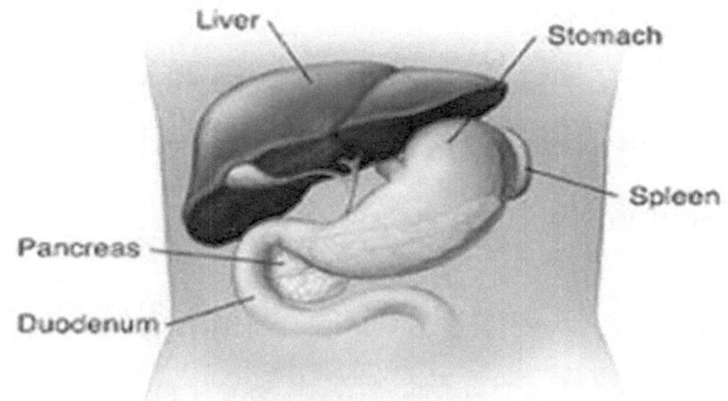

Diagram Showing the Pancreas

HOW COMMON IS DIABETES MELLITUS?

Diabetes has become a global pandemic that shows no signs of abating anytime soon, as its prevalence continues to increase worldwide.

According to the World Health Organization (WHO), there are currently 422 million people living with diabetes worldwide, and sadly, 1.5 million people die each year as a direct result of the disease. Sadly, those living in middle- and low-income countries are disproportionately affected by this epidemic.

Moreover, in 2021, The International Diabetes Federation (IDF) puts the figure of adults (20-79 years) living with diabetes at 537 million, projected to rise to 643 million and 783 million by 2030 and 2045 respectively. Over 1 million children and adolescents are also living with Diabetes.

According to the IDF, 24 million adults have diabetes in the IDF African Region, out of which 11.2 million are in Nigeria. This prevalence in the African Region is projected to increase to 33 million by 2030 and 55 million by 2045.

Types of Diabetes Mellitus

Diabetes Mellitus can be classified into two main types: primary and secondary. Primary DM occurs when the pancreas has a problem with insulin secretion or when the body cannot effectively utilise insulin. Primary DM can be further subdivided into: ***Type 1 and Type 2 Diabetes Mellitus.***

Type 1 Diabetes Mellitus

Type 1 diabetes occurs when the pancreas fails to produce insulin, resulting in a condition known as Absolute Insulin Deficiency. This is often due to a combination of genetic predisposition and autoimmune conditions, where the body's immune system attacks its own pancreas, leading to its destruction.

Type 1 diabetes typically develops before age 30, although it can occur at any age. There are various potential triggers, including:

a) Viruses

b) Toxins

c) Stress, either physical or emotional.

d) Dietary factors.

e) Although controversial, early cessation of breastfeeding is also considered a possible trigger.

f) Born by Caesarean section.

SYMPTOMS OF TYPE 1 DIABETES MELLITUS

a) Excessive urination

b) Increased thirst leading to excessive water consumption

c) Excessive hunger leading to overeating

d) Weight loss

e) Body Mass Index (BMI), which is a weight-to-height ratio, of less than 25kg/m2

f) Easy fatigability.

g) Bedwetting

h) Elevated Random Blood Sugar greater than 11.1mmol/l or 200mg/dl

i) Ketosis, which is the accumulation of a chemical substance called ketones and can lead to a medical emergency known as Diabetic Ketoacidosis (DKA). DKA involves high blood glucose levels, breathing difficulties, severe dehydration, low blood pressure, and even loss of consciousness.

NB: The first three symptoms are the general symptoms of DM

The treatment for type 1 diabetes involves following a daily insulin regimen, monitoring your blood sugar levels regularly, and maintaining a healthy lifestyle. People with Type 1 Diabetes must take their insulin daily, as without it, they can experience life-threatening complications within days or weeks.

Therefore, if you have been diagnosed with Type 1 Diabetes, taking your insulin as prescribed is essential. Additionally, it's advisable to self-monitor your blood sugar levels regularly to ensure they stay within a safe range.

TYPE 2 DIABETES MELLITUS

Type 2 diabetes occurs due to a relative insulin deficiency, meaning that the pancreas is not producing enough insulin or the body's cells are not responding properly to the insulin (known as insulin resistance), despite normal or increased insulin levels.

This type of diabetes is usually seen in people over 30, but it is becoming increasingly common in children and adolescents due to the rise in obesity and unhealthy diets. Genetic predisposition and lifestyle factors also play a significant role in developing type 2 diabetes.

If you have any of the following, you may be at an increased risk of developing type 2 diabetes:

a) Obesity or being overweight, indicated by a BMI greater than 25kg/m2. This can cause insulin resistance, which can lead to type 2 diabetes.

b) Leading a sedentary lifestyle.

c) Having a family history of diabetes.

d) Having Metabolic Syndrome, which is a group of conditions that includes high blood pressure, high blood sugar, high blood cholesterol, and obesity, particularly with central tummy fat.

e) Advancing age, greater than 45 years.

f) Having a history of gestational diabetes.

g) Having blood sugar levels in the prediabetes range

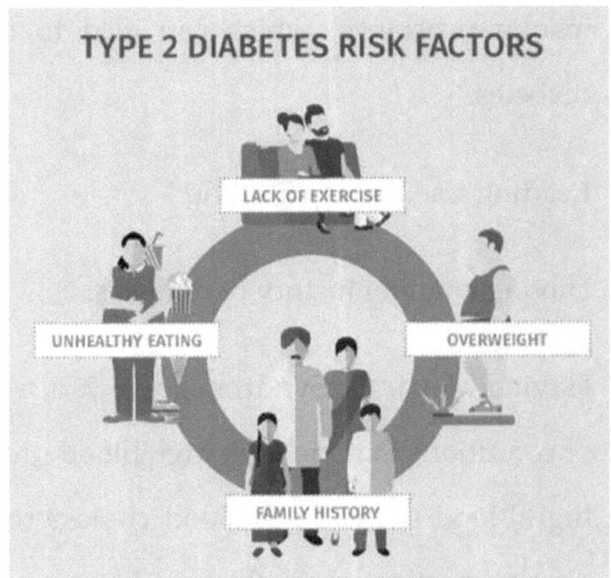

Picture Showing Risk Factors For Diabetes

SYMPTOMS OF TYPE 2 DM

The symptoms of Type 2 DM include the general symptoms of diabetes, as previously mentioned, including excessive urination, increased thirst leading to excessive water consumption, and excessive hunger leading to overeating. Additionally, other symptoms may include:

a) Recurrent infections, such as urinary tract infections, recurrent boils, vaginal candidiasis, and vaginal dryness in females

b) Weight gain or loss.

c) Blurry vision.

d) Tiredness.

e) Erectile dysfunction and low sex drive in men.

f) Poor wound healing.

g) Paresthesia and tingling in the hands and feet.

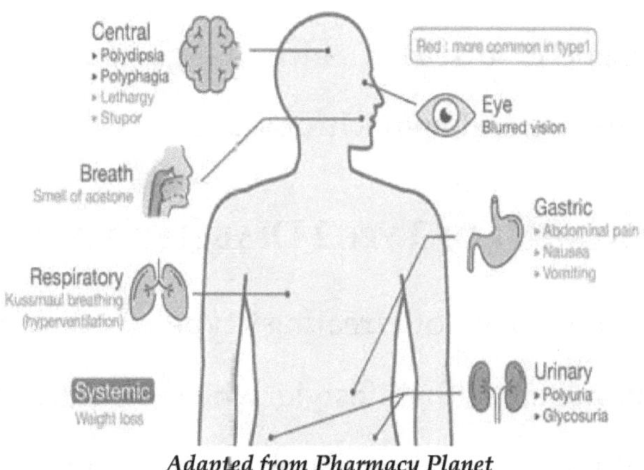

Adapted from Pharmacy Planet

SECONDARY DIABETES MELLITUS

This occurs when blood sugar levels are elevated due to other medical conditions. These conditions include:

a) Pancreatic diseases, such as chronic pancreatitis, pancreatic cancer, and cystic fibrosis.

b) Endocrine (hormonal) conditions, such as Cushing's syndrome, pheochromocytoma, and acromegaly.

c) Drug-induced conditions, caused by medications like thiazide, beta-blockers, and antipsychotics.

d) Genetic diseases, such as glycogen storage disease and hemochromatosis.

TREATMENT OF TYPE 2 DIABETES MELLITUS

The cornerstone of treating type 2 diabetes is maintaining a healthy lifestyle, which includes regular physical activity, healthy eating, maintaining a healthy weight, and avoiding smoking. However, in some cases, a healthy lifestyle may not be enough to control blood glucose levels in the long run. This is where medications called Oral Hypoglycaemic Agents (OHAs) come in.

OHAs are divided into different categories, each with its specific mode of action. These medications help to lower blood sugar levels through various mechanisms.

Metformin is typically the first medication prescribed to achieve the desired blood sugar control, and it may be combined with other types of medication as well. However, insulin may be required if oral hypoglycemic agents (OHAs) are insufficient to control blood glucose levels.

This occurs when there is treatment failure or when the pancreas is no longer producing insulin. It's important to understand that medication is necessary to support and complement the amount of insulin your pancreas produces.

Remember that each patient is unique, and your doctor has tailored your treatment plan accordingly. Avoid comparing your medication regimen to others, and never share your medication with others.

If you're travelling, inform your doctor and ensure you take enough drugs for the journey, and preferably you visit a doctor when you get to your destination.

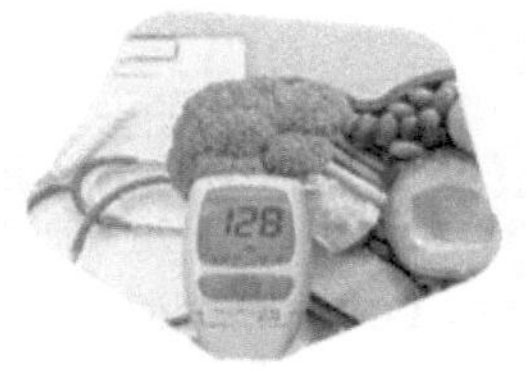

CHAPTER THREE

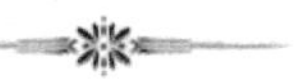

Diagnosis of Diabetes

"Diabetes may be a challenge, but it is not a definition"-Unknown

HOW IS DIABETES MELLITUS DIAGNOSED?

Diabetes can be diagnosed with or without the presence of symptoms. When symptoms are present, an elevated blood sugar level of Random Blood Sugar greater than or equal to 11.1mmol/l, Fasting Blood sugar of greater than or equal to 7.0mmol/l, or Glycated Haemoglobin (HbA1c) of greater than or equal to 6.5% is diagnostic of DM.

HbA1c provides an idea of your blood glucose levels over the past three months, making it useful for monitoring how you've responded to treatment during that time if you're currently receiving diabetes treatment.

However, more than one elevated blood glucose test is usually required when no symptoms exist. It's recommended that the same test be repeated for accuracy. If the results are normal, regular follow-up is needed.

If the type of diabetes is unclear, your doctor may request further blood tests, such as the Glutamic Acid Decarboxylase (GAD) Autoantibodies test, C-peptide test, or Ketone test. One or two of these tests can confirm if your diabetes is type 1.

DIFFERENT TYPES OF BLOOD SUGAR TESTS

1. Random Blood Sugar (RBS): This test measures your blood glucose levels at any time of the day without requiring you to fast. If your value is

above 200mg/dl or 11.1mmol/L, it may suggest or confirm diabetes.

2. Fasting Blood Sugar (FBS): This test is done after an overnight fast of 8-12 hours before you eat breakfast. Drinking water is allowed. Your fasting blood sugar level should be less than 100mg/dl or 5.6 mmol/L. If it falls between 108-125mg/dl(6.0-6.9mmol/L), it indicates prediabetes, while anything above 7.0mmol/L is suggestive or confirmatory of diabetes.

3. Two Hours Postprandial Blood Sugar (2HPP): This test measures your blood sugar level two hours after eating. Normal levels should be less than 7.8mmol/L or 140mg/dl. If it falls between 7.8-11.0mmol/L (140-199mg/dl), it indicates prediabetes, while anything above 11.1mmol/L or 200mg/dl may suggest or confirm diabetes.

4. Oral Glucose Tolerance Test (OGTT): This test involves taking a fasting blood sample in the

morning, followed by a 75g glucose drink. Another blood sample is taken two hours later to measure blood sugar levels. This test is used to screen for type 2 diabetes and gestational diabetes. Blood sugar levels above 11.1mmol/L are considered abnormal.

5. Glycated Haemoglobin (HbA1c): This test measures your average blood sugar level over the past three months.

   Normal levels are below 42mmol/mol (5.6%). Prediabetes is between 42-47mmol/mol (5.7-6.4%), while diabetes is above 48mmol/mol (6.5% and above).

Being honest with your healthcare provider is essential when undergoing these tests. Remember, the goal is not to make you diabetic but to detect it early and prevent complications.

WHO SHOULD GO FOR BLOOD SUGAR TESTING?

Diabetes is a stealthy disease that can develop without noticeable symptoms until it becomes a medical emergency. Sometimes it is only discovered during routine check-ups.

It is vital to get tested if:

a. You are experiencing any of the symptoms earlier mentioned.

b. You have a first-degree relative with diabetes.

c. You have high blood pressure and/or obesity.

d. You have given birth to a baby weighing 4.5kg (10 pounds) or more.

e. It is a part of your routine medical check-up.

WHY MUST YOU KNOW ABOUT DIABETES MELLITUS?

Diabetes Mellitus is a lifelong disease that can cause severe damage or complications to your body, both chronic (long-term) and acute (life-threatening emergencies). Some chronic complications, like heart attack, can lead to sudden death, while others, like stroke and chronic kidney disease, can drastically reduce the quality of life.

For people with type 1 Diabetes, insulin replacement is crucial for survival, as they may die within days or weeks without it. However, with insulin replacement, they can lead a normal life, although they are at risk of complications.

According to the World Health Organization (WHO), approximately 1.5 million people die of diabetes every year, and about 33% of those with Diabetes develop Diabetic Eye Disease, which is a leading cause of blindness.

Unfortunately, as the number of people living with diabetes is expected to rise, so is the occurrence of complications.

Therefore, knowing diabetes, how to prevent it if you are at risk, and managing it if you already have it, can empower you to lead a good and rewarding life. You can avert the complications mentioned above with the proper knowledge and approach to DM.

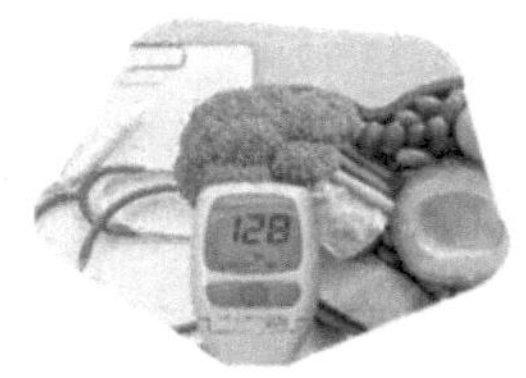

CHAPTER FOUR

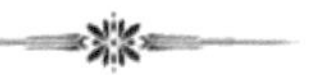

Diabetes Complications

"The diabetic patient must be educated to take care of himself, and to avoid the complications of the disease"-Bernhard Naunyn (1898)

Diabetes can cause significant damage to various parts of your body, including the brain, eyes, heart, blood vessels, kidneys, nerves, and more. These complications can be broadly classified into two categories: acute and chronic complications

ACUTE COMPLICATIONS

There are life-threatening emergencies that can arise from diabetes mellitus. Examples include:

a. Hyperosmolar Hyperglycaemic State (HHS): This usually occurs in type 2 diabetes and can be a life-threatening condition that presents with high blood sugar, extreme tiredness, and worsening symptoms of excessive urination, thirst, seizures, and coma. It can lead to death if not quickly managed.

b. Lactic Acidosis is the accumulation of acidic substances in the blood and can result in breathing problems and death.

c. Diabetic Ketoacidosis (DKA): This is the third acute complication and is usually seen in type 1 diabetes and can be life-threatening. People with type 1 diabetes may not know they have it until they develop this condition and are diagnosed for the first time.

   DKA occurs when there is insufficient insulin to move blood sugar into your cells for energy production. Thus, your liver resorts to other pathways, like breaking down fats and protein to generate energy. This breaking down of fats releases toxic substances called ketone bodies. And when these substances accumulate to dangerous levels, they lead to DKA.

It is a medical emergency and should be treated as such.

Symptoms include dry skin and mouth, fast and deep breathing, extreme tiredness, vomiting, fruit-smelling breath, seizures, and coma.

Possible triggers include missing insulin doses, infections such as urinary tract infection, chest infection, gastrointestinal infection, malaria, stroke or heart attack, trauma such as car accidents, and drugs like steroids.

The mainstay of treatment is administering rapidly-acting insulin and fluid and addressing other accompanying problems.

d. Hypoglycaemia (Hypo for short): This is when your blood sugar drops too low (usually below 4mmol/l or 70mg/dl). It usually occurs when a person with diabetes takes an overdose of sugar-lowering drugs, whether insulin or oral hypoglycemic agents (OHA).

It is a life-threatening condition that should be quickly and can be easily treated with a glucose-containing substance or drink.

Please note that it is crucial to seek medical attention immediately if any of these conditions arise, as timely intervention can prevent potentially fatal consequences.

HYPOGLYCAEMIC AWARENESS

Hypoglycemic awareness is the ability of a person with diabetes to recognise the symptoms of low blood sugar, especially when taking medication. It is essential because hypoglycemia can be life-threatening and needs to be promptly addressed when it arises.

Being aware of hypoglycemia helps you to take steps to manage low blood sugar when it happens.

Repeated hypoglycemic exposure can lead to a clinical condition called Impaired Hypoglycemic Awareness (IHA).

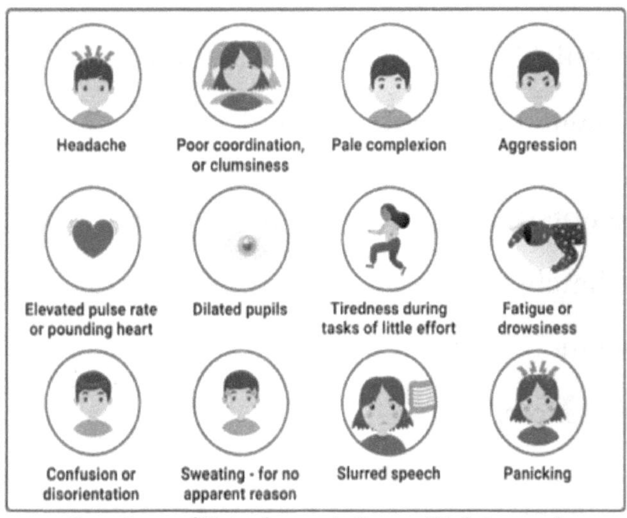

Symptoms of Hypoglycaemia Source: Diabetes.co.uk

This condition causes a decrease in the ability to recognize hypoglycemic symptoms and puts the individual at risk of severe hypoglycemia, which can result in death or a vegetative state.

Therefore, you may be experiencing hypoglycemia if you start:

a. Sweating

b. Feeling confused

c. Shaking

d. Becoming restless, nervous, or irritable

e. Feeling hungry

f. Having a fast heartbeat

g. Experiencing a headache or lack of concentration

When your blood sugar falls below normal, your body produces a surge of adrenaline which is responsible for the symptoms of hypoglycemia.

WHAT SHOULD YOU DO IF YOU DEVELOP HYPOGLYCEMIA?

To prevent fits or comas, it's important to treat hypoglycemia quickly. If you experience symptoms, use the 15-15 rule: consume 15g of fast-acting carbohydrate and check your blood sugar 15 minutes later. If it's still below 4mmol/l or 70mg/dl, have another 15g of carbohydrate and repeat the process until your blood sugar level is above 4mmol/l or 70mg/dl. Once your levels stabilise, eat a normal meal or snack to maintain your blood sugar levels.

Remember to keep track of the causes and symptoms of your hypo and discuss them with your healthcare provider to help prevent future occurrences.

Examples of fast-acting carbohydrates include glucose tablets or glucose D, small bottles of sugary drinks, and fruit juice.

If symptoms persist, seek medical attention immediately.

THE LONG TERM OR CHRONIC COMPLICATIONS OF DIABETES

The Long-term complications of Diabetes include:

a. Diabetic Eye Disease, which can lead to visual disturbances and blindness. Diabetes can cause cataracts and glaucoma, which can eventually result in blindness.

b. Cerebrovascular diseases such as stroke and dementia.

c. Cardiovascular Disease, including heart disease, heart attack, and blood vessel disease.

d. Diabetic Kidney Disease, which can impair kidney function and lead to chronic kidney disease.

e. Nerve Disease, which can cause numbness, tingling, and other sensations.

f. Erectile Dysfunction and reduced libido.

g. Diabetic Foot Ulcer.

It's essential to manage diabetes properly to prevent these chronic complications from developing over time.

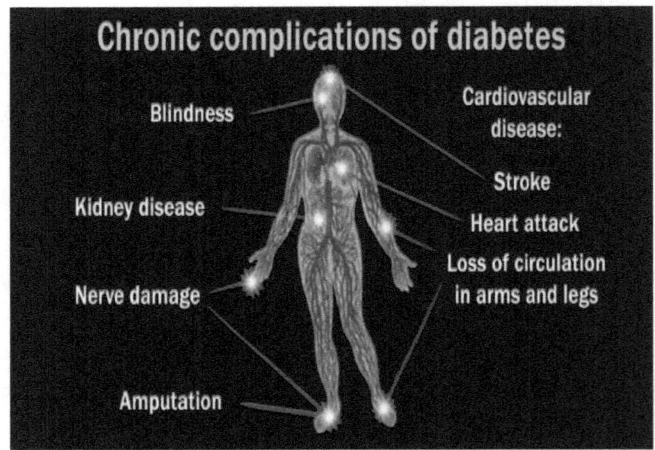

Picture showing chronic complications of diabetes. Courtesy of YogaTute Health

DIABETIC FOOT DISEASE

Diabetes can sometimes damage your nerves, causing pain, numbness, and paraesthesia. On the other hand, you may lose sensation in your feet as a result of nerve damage and be unaware of wounds or objects in your shoes or socks. This can lead to sores and infection.

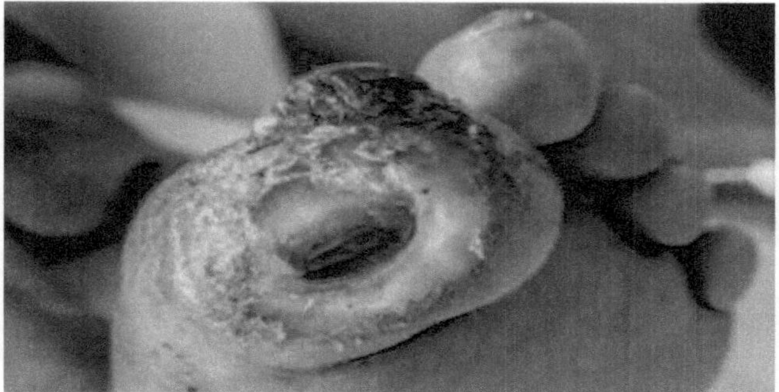

Picture of Diabetic Foot Ulcer. Adapted from Dermnet

Additionally, diabetes can reduce blood flow to your feet, which can cause ulcers to form or prevent existing ones from healing. If an ulcer or infection becomes severe, it can progress to gangrene.

In cases where treatment is ineffective, gangrene or a non-healing foot ulcer may require amputation of your foot or toe to prevent the infection from spreading to other parts of your body and save your life.

WHAT CAN YOU DO TO PREVENT DIABETES FOOT ULCER?

Your diabetic management plan should include foot care, and there are several things you can do to prevent the development of ulcers in your feet. These include:

a. Daily foot examination: You may have problems in your foot but not feel any pain, so it's essential to check your feet daily for any sores. Remember to examine your feet for cuts, red spots, blisters, and calluses in the evening when you remove your shoes. Also, check between your toes for any cracks or sores and examine the underside of your foot for any growth, warmth, or redness.

    If you're at an increased risk of developing sores, your doctor may recommend measuring the temperature of different parts of the skin on your foot. An increase in temperature in any part may signal the development of an ulcer or blister.

b. Daily washing and drying of your feet in warm water: Avoid using hot water to prevent unintended skin burning. Make sure to dry the spaces between your toes and apply cornstarch or talcum powder to keep them less moist and to avoid infection.

c. Avoid extremes of heat on your extremities, especially if you have nerve problems: You should not use heating pads on your body and keep away from open fires. If you're at the beach, wear shoes on hot surfaces.

Wear boots in the winter or during the harmattan period to keep your feet warm and dry. Wear socks to keep your feet warm if they become cold in bed.

d. If you have dry skin, it is recommended that you apply lubricants such as urea or salicylates to your legs. However, do not apply lubricants to the spaces between your toes, as moisture can lead to infection.

e. To keep blood flowing in your legs, try to elevate them when you are sitting and wiggle your shoes throughout the day to enhance blood flow in your feet and legs. Engaging in activities such as walking, yoga, dancing, biking, or swimming can also help to improve blood flow in your lower extremities

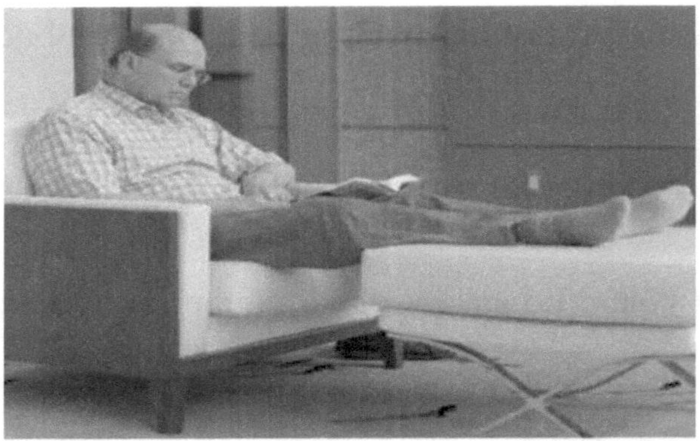

Putting up your feet while sitting in this manner ensures blood circulation.
Source: NIDDK

f. Be careful when cutting your toenails to avoid injuring your toes. Avoid rounding the corners or cutting into the corners of your nails in a V-shape. Instead, cut straight across to prevent any injuries

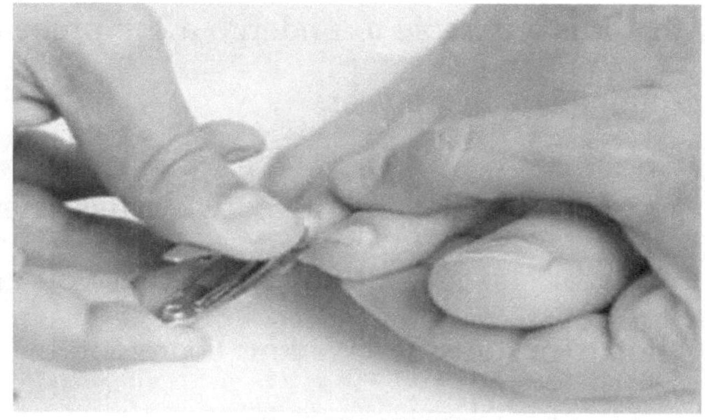

Adapted from NIDDK

g. Ensure your healthcare provider checks your feet at every clinic visit. Take off your shoes and socks during the examination to remind them to check your feet thoroughly. The examination may include:

i.   Checking for ulcers, redness, discharge, or warmth

ii. ii. Noting any changes in the shape of your legs and feet

iii. Evaluating your ability to feel pain, vibration, and position

iv. Assessing the pulses in your feet

Note that it is advisable to undergo a comprehensive foot examination once a year.

> h. When it comes to footwear, it is essential to wear shoes at all times, whether you are at home or outside. Walking barefoot or only wearing socks can be dangerous as you could step on something and hurt yourself without feeling any pain until it's too late. Also, check inside your shoes and socks for any potential threats.

Consider the following when choosing footwear:

i. Wear shoes that fit properly and protect your feet.

ii. ii. Athletic shoes are a good choice for daily activities as they fit well and provide comfort.

iii. Buy your footwear at the end of the day when your feet are likely to be the largest to ensure the best fit.

iv. Avoid high heels or pointed toes, as they put too much pressure on your toes.

v. you may need special orthotic shoes if you have deformed feet.

vi. Ensure your shoes have an enclosed frontal part to prevent toe injury.

vii. When wearing a new pair of shoes, wear them briefly and check your feet for any soreness.

Remember, taking care of your feet is crucial in preventing complications from diabetes.

WHEN SHOULD YOU CONSULT YOUR HEALTH CARE GIVER FOR FOOT PROBLEMS?

It is advisable to promptly consult your healthcare provider if you observe any of the following:

a. Redness, warmth, or pain on any of your feet, as these could be signs of an infection.

b. A blister, bruise, or cut on your foot that shows no signs of healing after a few days.

c. A foot infection that is turning black and has an offensive odour could be the onset of gangrene.

Your doctor may refer you to a foot specialist if necessary.

DIABETES AND YOUR EYESIGHT- HOW DOES IT IMPACT YOUR EYEGLASS PRESCRIPTION?

You may be aware that blurry vision is one of the symptoms of diabetes, but what you may not know is that diabetes can cause subtle changes to your eyes that can affect your eyeglass prescription. Diabetes can affect every part of the eye, and these changes can occur before you are diagnosed with diabetes.

Diabetes can cause small haemorrhages, cataracts, dry eyes, glaucoma, diabetic eye disease, and swelling of the part of the eye responsible for reading and driving.

It's important to take care of your eyes and have regular eye exams if you have diabetes.

How Does Diabetes Affect Your Eyeglass Prescription?

The eye is a complex organ with many tiny blood vessels. Diabetes and high blood pressure can cause damage to these vessels, making it essential to take care of your eyes.

When your blood glucose level rises, the lens in your eyes can swell up and cause changes in your vision. You may become farsighted or nearsighted, or if you already have these conditions, diabetes can make them worse. This happens because of the fluctuations in your blood sugar levels.

Suppose you need prescription eyeglasses to correct your vision. In that case, getting an eye exam and ensuring your blood sugar level is normal before you get the right eyeglass prescription is important. This is because changes in your blood sugar level can cause changes in your vision and affect your eyeglass prescription. If you experience any change in your vision, do not ignore them or see them as a sign of tiredness. It is crucial to see your healthcare provider for appropriate action.

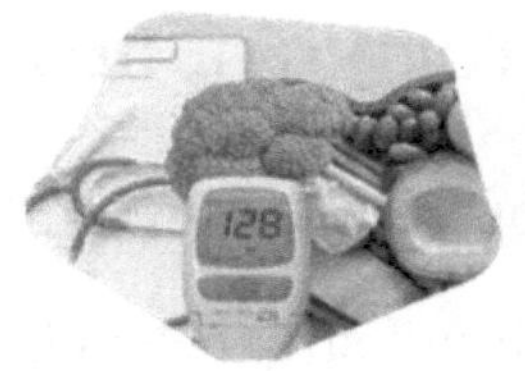

CHAPTER FIVE

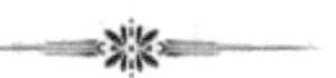

Self-Management Of Diabetes

DEFINITION

Self-management of diabetes refers to the activities and behaviour patterns adopted by a person living with diabetes to manage their condition, with a view to achieve control and prevent or delay complications. This includes monitoring blood glucose levels and involves the following:

SELF-MONITORING OF BLOOD GLUCOSE

Self-monitoring of blood glucose is the practice of checking one's blood sugar levels at any time and place, whether at home, school, or work.

This is crucial because it allows people with diabetes and their healthcare providers to observe how their blood sugar levels change throughout the day and adjust their treatment plan to optimise blood sugar control. This brings us to the practice of home blood glucose monitoring.

HOME BLOOD GLUCOSE MONITORING

A home blood glucose test is a simple, affordable, and convenient way to check and monitor your blood sugar levels to prevent complications. It allows you to assess how well you are managing your blood glucose.

Regularly checking your blood glucose levels is one of the best ways to manage your diabetes. It helps you and your healthcare provider understand your condition better and how foods, exercise, and medications impact your blood glucose.

In addition, home glucose monitoring can help you recognise when your blood sugar levels are too high or too low, helping to prevent emergencies such as hypo and DKA. So, it's an important tool in managing your diabetes and staying healthy

HOW IS HOME BLOOD GLUCOSE MONITORING DONE?

Home blood glucose monitoring is an essential part of diabetes management. It involves using a home glucose test kit, including a small glucometer, specialised strips, and a lancet.

With this kit, you can check your blood sugar levels regularly and adjust your diet or medication accordingly, helping you to maintain optimal glucose control and prevent complications.

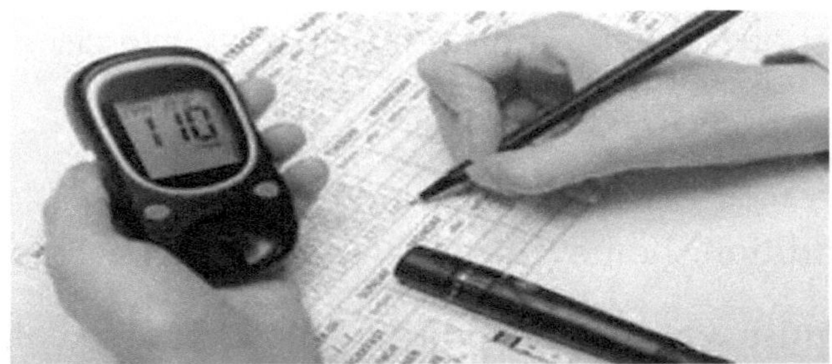

Diagrams showing a glucometer, glucometer strip, log book, and a needle-holding device

It is advisable to keep a record of the food you eat to observe the patterns of your blood glucose. Remember that an elevated blood sugar after a meal, whether you eat high- or low-carbohydrate food, may indicate that your body is not handling blood glucose well after eating.

Glucometers are available in different sizes and at varying costs. Some have additional technologies to meet specific needs, such as added memory storage to enhance the glucometer's memory, a backlit screen to help you see clearly in low light, an audio feature to assist those with hearing impairment. And, preloaded strips to help those with hand problems.

TIPS FOR CHOOSING A GLUCOMETER

To successfully measure blood glucose levels, you will need a blood kit, which includes a glucometer (blood sugar monitor), testing strips, and a lancet or small needle to obtain blood. Considering the cost of strips and glucometer is essential since you will need several testing strips for the exercise. Here are some other things to keep in mind:

a. glucose testing Look for size and portability that makes it easy to carry around.

b. Check if your insurance covers some glucometer kits.

c. Consider a glucometer with automatic coding to avoid coding the result of each test.

d. Look for a glucometer that has storage capability.

e. Choose a monitor requiring a smaller blood sample volume, as it makes pricking less painful.

PREPARING FOR BLOOD GLUCOSE MEASUREMENT

Before measuring your blood sugar level, ensure you have the following:

a. Strips that have not expired.

b. A lancet or any other finger-prick tool

c. A glucometer

d. Alcohol swabs

e. A bandage in case bleeding continues after pricking your finger.

HOW TO MEASURE YOUR BLOOD SUGAR LEVEL

a. Carefully wash your hands to prevent infecting the pricking site. You can do this using an alcohol swab or warm, soapy water. In any case, allow your hand to dry before you start testing.

b. Remove a strip from its container and insert it into the glucometer. Ensure to wholly and immediately close the container to avoid chemical reactions that can tamper with the strips.

c. Use a lancet tc prick the side of your finger to get a drop of blood. Using the side of the finger instead of the tip decreases discomfort. Read the manual of your kit, as some allow you to draw blood from other parts of the body.

d. Wipe off the first drop of blood and then gently squeeze the finger to allow a drop of blood into the test spot of the strip.

e. Finally, allow the glucometer to analyse and display your blood glucose on its screen.

f. Record your blood glucose in a logbook or notebook after each test, noting the time you performed the test.

g. Stop the bleeding by firmly applying a gauze or cotton wool ball to the lanced area.

h. Dispose of the strips, lancet, and other tools you used into a safety box.

Note: Do not use someone else's lancet or glucose monitor to protect yourself from contracting blood-borne infections such as HIV, Hepatitis B, or Hepatitis C.

CONTINUOUS GLUCOSE MONITORING (CGM)

Continuous glucose monitoring is a technology that makes it easier for you to keep tab of your blood sugar levels throughout 24 hours a day. You can track your glucose levels anytime in an instant.

CGM helps you to observe the fluctuations in your glucose levels over a few hours or days to track patterns. By viewing your glucose levels in the present moment, you can use this information to make better-informed decisions about how to balance your food intake, physical activity, and medication regimen throughout the day.

HOW DOES A CONTINUOUS GLUCOSE MONITOR FUNCTION?

A CGM works through a tiny sensor inserted under your skin, usually on your belly or arm. The sensor measures your interstitial glucose level, which is the glucose found in the fluid between the cells. The sensor tests glucose every few minutes. A transmitter wirelessly sends the information to a monitor.

The monitor may be part of an insulin pump or a separate device, which you might carry in a pocket or purse. Some CGMs send information directly to a smartphone or tablet.

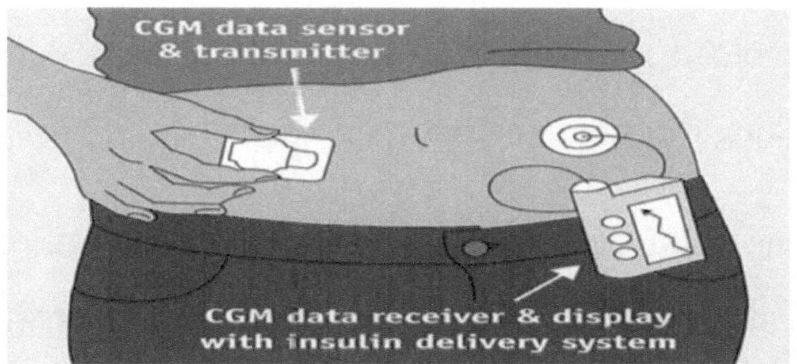

A tiny under the skin checks glucose. A transmitter sends data to a receiver. The CGM sensor CGM receiver may be part of an insulin pump, as shown here, or a separate device such as a smartphone. Adapted from NIDDK Website

FEATURES OF CGM

CGMs have unique features that make them stand out. They are designed to continuously monitor glucose levels in real-time, regardless of what you are doing, be it showering, working, exercising, or sleeping.

These devices often have special capabilities that work alongside the glucose readings, such as an alarm that alerts you when your glucose level goes too low or too high.

Additionally, you can keep track of your meals, physical activities, and medications on the CGM device, along with your glucose levels. You can download the data to a computer or smart device, making it easier to monitor glucose trends.

Some CGM models can also send information directly to a designated person's smartphone, such as a parent, partner, or caregiver. For instance, if a child's glucose drops to a dangerous level overnight, the CGM can be set to wake up a parent in the next room.

THE REQUIREMENTS OF CGM

To use a CGM, there are certain requirements that you need to follow. You may need to check the CGM twice a day by testing a drop of blood on a standard glucose meter to ensure the accuracy of both devices' readings.

Additionally, you will have to replace the CGM sensor every 3 to 7 days, depending on the specific model.

When the CGM alarm goes off about high or low blood glucose, it is important to take appropriate action for your safety. You should follow your treatment plan to bring your glucose levels into the target range, or seek assistance if necessary.

ADVANTAGES OF USING CGM

Using a CGM system can provide several benefits compared to a standard blood glucose meter, including:

a. improved daily management of glucose levels

b. a reduction in low blood glucose emergencies

c. a decreased need for finger sticks

HOW TO INTERPRET YOUR BLOOD GLUCOSE LEVEL

Please note that each person's blood glucose levels can vary depending on factors such as general health, age, and weight. Therefore, discussing with your doctor to determine your target values is important.

However, the recommended ranges for blood glucose levels are as follows:

a. Fasting: 80-130mg/dl (4.4-7.2mmol/l)

b. Two hours after a meal: below 180mg/dl (< 10mmol/L)

c. At bedtime: less than 120mg/dl (6.7mmol/l)

d. HbA1c: less than 7%

These values are based on when the tests are carried out, and they serve as a guide to help manage your blood glucose levels effectively

What If You Consistently Have High Home Blood Sugar

Consult your doctor if you repeatedly record abnormally high home blood glucose levels. Your doctor may advise you to make lifestyle changes, take medications, or both.

However, it's important to note that some factors can affect your home blood glucose levels. Therefore, do not panic if you notice that your blood sugar is not within the targeted range. These factors include:

a. Illness or infection.

b. The type and timing of your meals.

c. Your medications.

d. Your hormone levels.

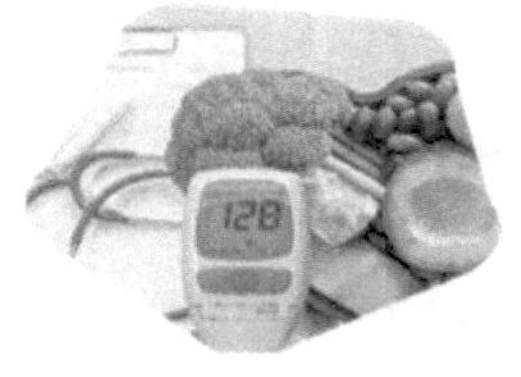

CHAPTER SIX

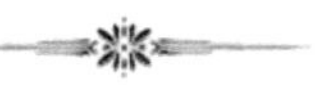

Insulin Therapy

"The discovery of insulin was the fruit of both human compassion and scientific genius"-Frederick Banting

INSULIN

There are misconceptions about insulin injections, as many people assume that being prescribed insulin means their condition is severe. However, the goal of insulin is to control blood sugar, and it does not always indicate that blood sugar levels have become unmanageable.

For individuals with type 1 diabetes, Insulin is often the best treatment in addition to a healthy lifestyle.

With type 2 diabetes, insulin may be required depending on how well the pancreas functions.

In general, insulin may be necessary for:

a. Type 1 diabetes

b. Diabetic emergencies such as DKA or HHS

c. Sepsis, or blood infection

d. Critically ill patients, such as those with heart attacks

e. Surgical procedures

f. Uncontrolled diabetes during pregnancy

g. Diabetic individuals who wish to become pregnant

h. Diabetic foot ulcers.

Cooperating with your doctor if you are prescribed Insulin is vital.

Remember that Insulin is only available in injectable form, but this does not mean your condition is severe if it is recommended for you.

TYPES OF INSULIN

There are different types of insulin based on how fast they work, their peak time, and duration of action. These types of Insulin include rapid-acting, short-acting, intermediate-acting, and long-acting.

a. **Rapid-acting Insulin:** it works within 15 minutes of injection, peaks at 2 hours, and lasts 2-4 hours. It controls blood sugar levels during or shortly after a meal. It's important to note that rapid-acting Insulin is clear and should not be overdosed to prevent hypoglycemia.

   Examples of rapid-acting Insulin include Aspart, Glulisine, and Lispro.

b. **Short-acting Insulin:** Short-acting Insulin (also known as regular Insulin) is similar to rapid-acting insulin, but its onset of action is slower. It takes about 15 to 30 minutes to start working. It reaches its maximum level (peak) at in 2-3 hours, and lasts 3-6 hours. Due to its slower onset of action, it can be taken before a meal.

It's worth noting that this type of Insulin is also clear in colour.

Examples include Actrapid, Humulin S, and Insuman Rapid

c. **Intermediate-acting Insulin:** Intermediate-acting Insulin starts working within the two hour of injection and lasts for about seven hours, after a period of peak activity. It is often taken with short-acting Insulin and should be taken once or twice a day.

This type of Insulin appears cloudy, and it is essential to gently invert it ten times until it is well mixed and turns white or milky in colour.

Examples of intermediate-acting Insulin include Insulintard and Humulin NPH

d. **Long-acting Insulin:** These are steadily released Insulins that can last in the system for up to 24 hours at a stretch. They are usually taken at night or in the morning. So, you only need to take it once a day. The risk of hypo is reduced with the use of long-acting insulin.

Their examples include Determir, Glargine, and Lantus.

e. **Ultra-long-acting Insulin:** This type does not peak and can last 36 hours in your system. An example is Degludec (Tresiba)

Kindly note that you should store your insulin inside your fridge away from sunlight. This ensures its efficacy is maintained, as temperature can break down insulin and make it lose its potency.

ADMINISTRATION OF INSULIN

Insulin can be administered through a syringe, Insulin pump, Insulin pen, or in powder form through inhalation. An Insulin pump is set to release a small amount of Insulin continuously, and if you need extra, you can adjust the pump accordingly.

INSULIN PEN

Insulin pens are preloaded with Insulin, allowing you to deliver the required insulin dose to the fatty layer under your skin with a thin, almost painless needle. Giving Insulin through an insulin pen is more reliable, simple, and convenient than using a syringe.

There are two different types of Insulin pens, and they are reusable and disposable. Reusable allows you to replace the Insulin cartridge once it is exhausted while you keep changing the pen needle each time you inject yourself.

Disposable type does not allow you the luxury of replacement. It contains a prefilled cartridge, which you discard once exhausted.

The one you will use will typically depend on the Insulin units you need per time.

EXPLAINING THE DIFFERENT PARTS OF INSULIN PEN

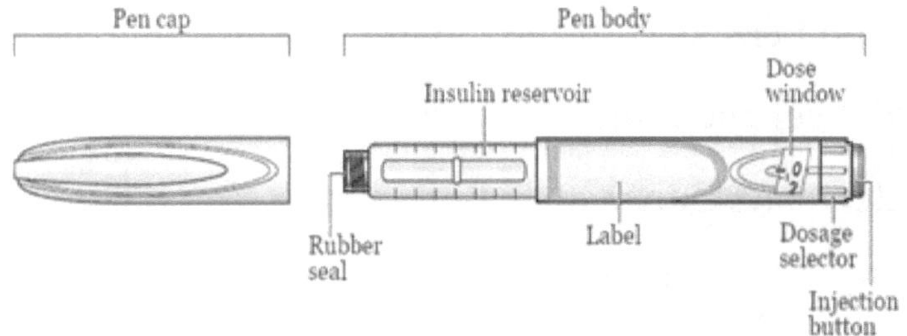

Adapted from Memorial Sloan Kettering Cancer Center.

Insulin pens typically come with different Insulin medications, but the fundamental parts remain the same. A basic insulin pen consists of two parts- a pen body and a pen cap.

Pen body: This part includes:

a. Injection button: Used to push Insulin in by pressing it.

b. Dosage selector: Dialed to set the right amount of Insulin required.

c. Dose window: Shows the amount or unit of Insulin dialed, signaled by an arrow that points directly to the selected units.

d. Insulin reservoir: Contains Insulin and is usually transparent, allowing the user to see how much insulin is left in the pen.

e. Label: Displays the Insulin type and expiry date.

f. Rubber seal: Junction between the pen body and pen cap.

HOW TO KEEP AN INSULIN PEN

Excessive heat, cold, or sunlight can damage the insulin in your insulin pen. Therefore, it is essential to know how to store it properly.

Here are some tips:

a. Store your unused, new Insulin pen in the refrigerator. However, avoid placing it at the back of the fridge to prevent it from freezing.

b. Once you start using your Insulin pen, keep it at room temperature, which should be below 86 degrees Fahrenheit or 30 degrees Celsius.

c. If you are going out in hot weather, protect your insulin pen from getting too hot by keeping it in an insulated bag or something similar to keep it cool.

d. Always remember to replace the insulin pen cap after use.

Typically, you will use your insulin pen for 7 to 28 days. However, discard it once it expires.

WHEN TO GIVE INSULIN INJECTION

When to inject your insulin depends on the type of Insulin you use.

For example:

a. If you are using rapid-acting Insulin, inject it about 15 minutes before a meal or take it shortly after a meal. Do not inject this type of insulin more often than 4 hours in between unless you are told otherwise by a healthcare professional. Injecting it less than four hours apart is risky because your blood sugar can crash too fast below normal.

b. If the type of insulin you are using is long-acting, use it at the same time of the day, whether morning or evening. However, abide by the instructions of your doctor.

INSULIN INJECTION SITES

There are various sites in the body where insulin can be injected, but the best site is the abdomen. Insulin is readily absorbed here, and it is also the most accessible site for self-injection.

Here are some tips on where to inject insulin:

a. Your belly, except for around 5cm from your belly button. This is the best site to use for rapid-acting insulin.

b. The outer and upper thigh. This site is best used for long-acting insulin.

c. The back aspect of your arms. However, you will need someone to assist you if you are using this site.

d. The upper part of your buttocks

Insulin injection sites

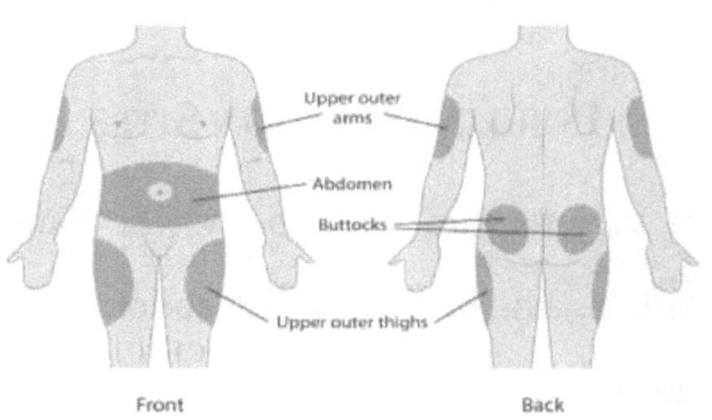

Insulin Injection Sites

Endeavour to keep record of the site you use, and ensure that you use you change the site with every injection. In the same injection site, leaving a space of about 2.5cm from the last injection point is advisable.

HOW TO INJECT INSULIN WITH INSULIN PEN

Insulin should be injected into the fatty layer under the skin, not the muscle. Observe the following steps when you are using insulin:

a. If you're using a new insulin pen, take it out of the refrigerator before use.

b. Check the expiry date and insulin type to ensure it's still valid.

c. Roll the insulin between your palms to mix it.

d. Wash your hands with soap and water, or use an alcohol swab.

e. Attach a new needle to the pen.

f. Remove the needle cap.

g. Dial the required dose.

h. Use your thumb and fingers to pick up and raise a fold of skin at the injection site.

i. Insert the needle at a 45-degree angle and inject the insulin into the fatty layer under the skin.

j. Hold the insulin pen in place for about 15 to 30 seconds after injecting to ensure maximum dose delivery.

k. Dispose of the needle in a sharps container.

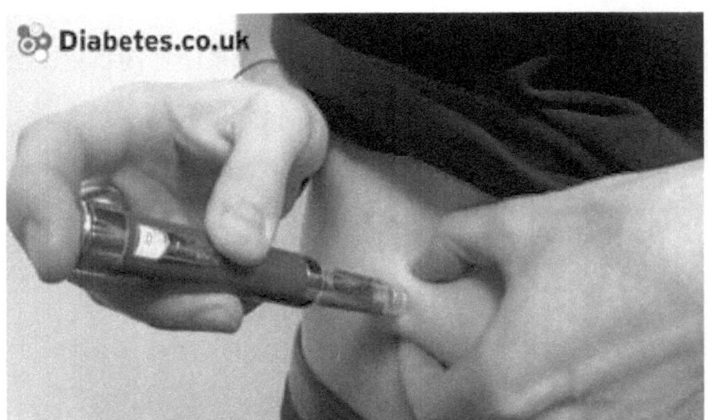

Diagram Showing How To Inject Insulin

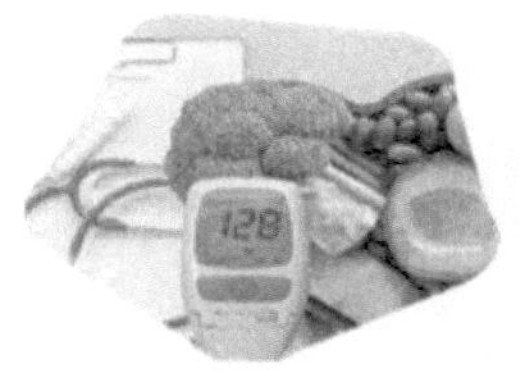

CHAPTER SEVEN

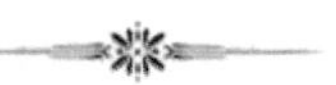

Prevention of Diabetes Complications

To prevent complications, it is important to control your blood sugar within acceptable limits.

The recommended schedules include:

1. Daily blood sugar checks

2. Visiting your doctor every 3-6 months to:

    a. Check your blood sugar levels and glycated hemoglobin.

    b. Examine injection sites if you are on insulin.

    c. Check your feet for any signs of diabetic foot disease.

3. Annual check-ups to:

    a. Monitor your cholesterol levels.

    b. Examine your eyes.

    c. Screen for diabetic kidney disease with a microalbuminuria test.

It is important to note that your specific schedule will depend on how well-controlled your glucose levels are, as there is no one-size-fits-all approach.

THE ABCS OF DIABETES MANAGEMENT

Being aware of your diabetes ABCs can help you focus on achieving and maintaining target values for your blood glucose levels, blood pressure, and cholesterol. By reaching your ABC goals, you can control your diabetes and prevent complications such as stroke, heart attack, and other vascular issues.

A stands for HbA1c or A1c

A blood glucose test measuring your average blood sugar level over the previous three months. The full name of the test is glycated haemoglobin or glycohaemoglobin test.

Haemoglobin is the component of your red blood cells that carries oxygen around your body. Glucose also attaches to haemoglobin, so the A1C test measures the amount of haemoglobin with attached glucose to reveal your blood glucose level over the last three months.

A1C is reported as a percentage, and the higher the percentage, the higher your blood glucose has been over the past twelve weeks. For people living with diabetes, the HbA1C goal should be less than 7%.

Be sure to discuss with your healthcare provider what your goal should be, and your doctor may recommend that you do this test twice a year.

B means Blood pressure

The target blood pressure should be below 140/80 mmHg. The higher your blood pressure, the harder your heart works, leading to complications. Therefore, have your blood pressure checked at every doctor's visit or whenever you have the opportunity.

C is for Cholesterol

You have different types of cholesterol in your blood, but they can be classified as either 'good' or 'bad'. HDL (High-Density Lipoprotein) represents the good cholesterol, while LDL (Low-density Lipoprotein) represents the bad cholesterol.

The bad type, LDL, can accumulate and narrow your blood vessels, leading to stroke or heart attack. However, the good cholesterol, HDL, helps to eliminate the bad ones from your system and prevent the adverse effects of the bad cholesterol.

Your target goals should be as follows:

a. LDL (bad) cholesterol should be less than 100mg/dl.

b. HDL (good) cholesterol should be above 40mg/dl for men and 50mg/dl for women.

c. Triglyceride levels should be less than 150mg/dl

Getting your cholesterol level checked at least once a year. Be advised that these values may need to be modified based on your parameters. So, always work alongside your healthcare provider.

Overall, it is essential to discuss your ABCs with your doctor to determine what your target numbers should be and what steps you can take to achieve healthy cholesterol parameters

S means Stop Smoking

Quitting smoking is crucial for those with diabetes, as smoking can damage blood vessels and increase the risk of cardiovascular complications like stroke and heart attack. It's important to note that E-cigarettes are not a safer alternative.

By quitting smoking or never starting, you can:

a. Reduce your risk of cardiovascular problems, diabetic eye issues, kidney disease, nerve damage, and amputation.

b. Improve blood flow throughout your body.

c. Potentially lower your blood pressure and cholesterol levels.

If you currently smoke, it's essential that you stop. Discuss with your healthcare provider about appropriate services to help you quit smoking

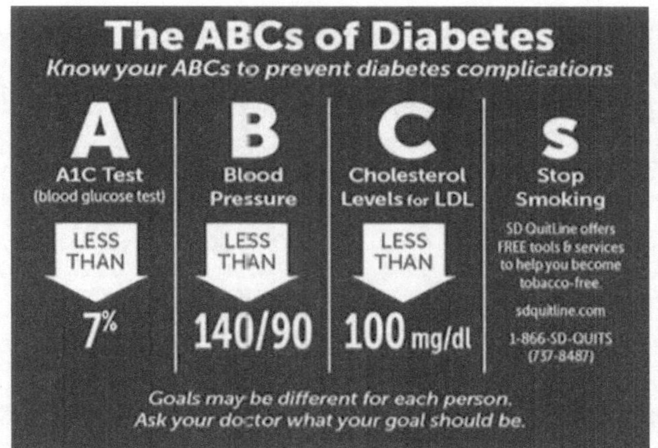

Source: Website of the State of South `Dakota department of health

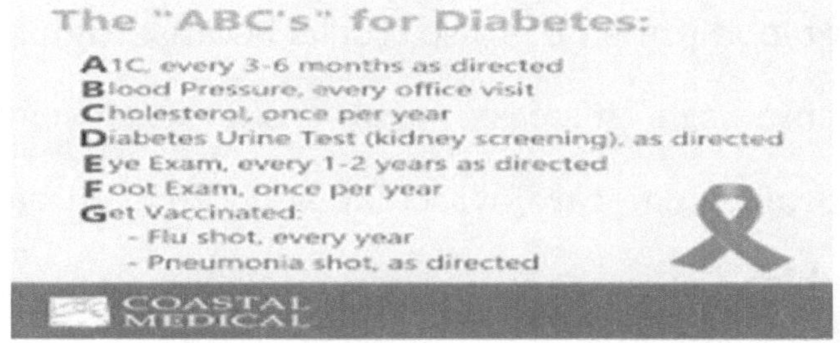

MEDICAL MEASURES TO DETECT COMPLICATIONS EARLY OR PREVENT COMPLICATIONS

Attending your follow-up appointments regularly is essential so your doctor can ask you questions about any complications you may have experienced or any medications you are taking.

During these appointments, your medications will be reviewed to determine whether to maintain the status quo, increase or reduce the dose, or introduce another medication based on your response to treatment.

Undergoing basic tests such as urine tests, kidney tests, cholesterol tests, and electrocardiograms (ECGs) can help detect chronic complications early. Monitoring your blood pressure is also crucial because high blood pressure can increase your risk of developing cerebrovascular, cardiovascular, and kidney disease. If your blood pressure is high, your doctor may prescribe medication to manage it.

Treating other medical conditions that coexist with diabetes, such as high blood cholesterol, is also important. Your doctor may prescribe aspirin to prevent blood clots. If you are obese, adopting a healthy lifestyle to lose weight is recommended. Metformin may be a suitable medication for individuals with both diabetes and obesity.

NON-MEDICAL MEASURES TO ACHIEVE CONTROL AND PREVENT COMPLICATIONS

a. Reduce Alcohol Consumption

Drinking alcohol beyond the recommended unit per week will not only damage your liver, but also put you at a higher risk of developing complications of diabetes. The recommended unit per week is 14 units, and there should be three days free of alcohol within the week.

So, not drinking alcohol above 14 units per week with three-free days in between will help prevent complications.

However, it is advisable to completely stop drinking alcohol if you have diabetes.

b. Regular Exercise

Regular exercise not only helps to control blood sugar but it also helps to prevent chronic complications of diabetes. By reducing insulin resistance and improving the body's ability to utilise blood sugar, exercise can keep blood glucose levels under control. It is vital to keep a glucose-containing substance with you while exercising in case you develop hypoglycemia.

To achieve maximum benefit, aerobic exercise (such as cycling, swimming, or jogging) should be combined with resistance exercise (such as sit-ups, push-ups, or squats), and sedentary lifestyle should be avoided.

Moderate aerobic exercise for 150 minutes per week, or 30 minutes per day for five days a week, is recommended. Alternatively, two sessions of 15 minutes per day can add up to the same total.

For vigorous exercise, 75 minutes per week, or 15 minutes per day for five days a week, is recommended.

Moderate exercise includes walking, swimming, cycling, and dancing, while vigorous exercise includes running, football, basketball, carrying heavy loads, and shoveling.

Suppose you have a knee condition like arthritis. In that case, weight-bearing activities may be challenging, so non-weight-bearing exercises like upper-extremity exercises or exercises in a lying position are recommended. Working with your doctor and exercise instructor is important to find the right exercise plan for you.

BENEFICIAL THINGS TO KNOW

If you have Diabetes Mellitus and experience any unusual symptoms, it is essential to see your doctor for evaluation.

Be aware of these specific symptoms and what they could mean for you as someone with DM:

a. Memory problems, clumsiness, or tremors may indicate brain complications such as dementia or cerebellar ataxia.

b. Sudden weakness in the face, arms or slurred speech may signal a stroke. Seek immediate medical attention if this occurs.

c. Visual disturbance could be a sign of developing diabetic eye disease.

d. Chest pain lasting longer than 15 minutes, chest pain that spreads to your neck, jaw, or shoulder, and palpitations may indicate heart disease or a heart attack.

It is worth noting that people with diabetes may not experience typical chest pain due to nerve damage that affects pain perception. This is known as Silent Chest. However, they may still experience palpitations, shortness of breath, sweating, or vomiting.

e. Pain in the calf muscles while walking that is relieved by rest may signal damage to blood vessels.

f. Numbness, paresthesia, a peppery sensation in the body, feeling like walking on sand or wool, and erectile dysfunction may point to nerve damage, known as diabetic neuropathy.

g. Swollen feet or excessively foamy urine may mean diabetic kidney disease.

If you notice any of these symptoms, it is advisable you see your healthcare giver on time for discussion and evaluation.

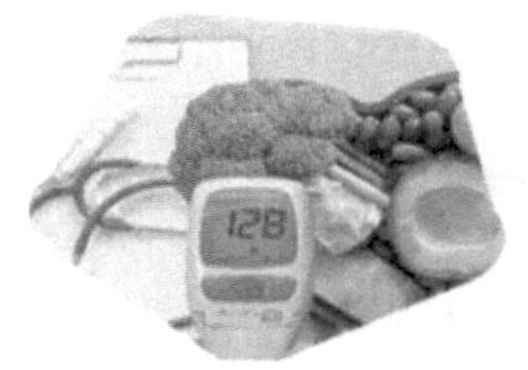

CHAPTER EIGHT

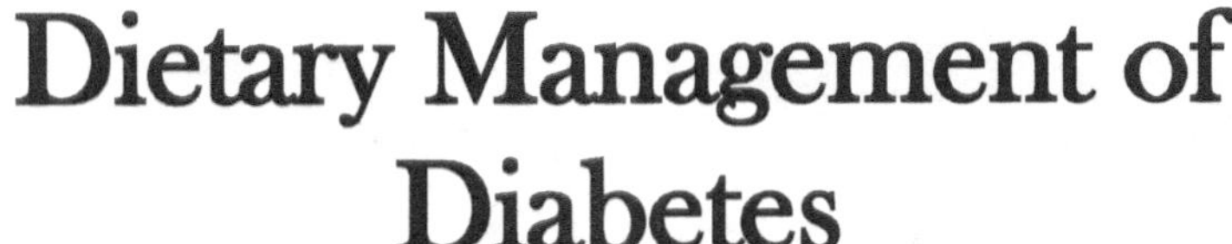

Dietary Management of Diabetes

"I have high blood sugars, and Type 2 diabetes is not going to kill me. But I just have to eat right, and exercise, and lose weight, and watch what I eat, and I will be fine for the rest of my life." — Tom Hanks.

With proper care, you can have a delicious and nutritious diet without having to cut out sugar, despite what you may have been told or believed.

The importance of a healthy diet in managing diabetes cannot be overstated. It is a crucial aspect of diabetes management and should be determined by your doctor and dietitian. The type of food you eat, the quantity you consume, and when you eat all play a vital role in achieving the blood sugar levels recommended by your healthcare team.

Although it is common to feel overwhelmed by the many food restrictions, you will find that dietary restrictions are not as rigid as you might think. It's just a matter of discipline in maintaining the recommended food portions and substituting saturated fats with unsaturated fats.

Your dietitian will educate you based on your unique medical condition and recommend the daily required calories from carbohydrates, proteins, and fats, considering your age, gender, weight, height, and physical activity level.

The benefits of dietary modifications in managing diabetes include the following:

a. It helps to keep your ABC within the range recommended by your doctor.

b. It enables you to maintain a healthy weight or lose weight, thereby improving your body's insulin sensitivity.

c. It helps in preventing or delaying the onset of complications.

What Foods Can You Eat?

The bedrock of the dietary plan for you is to eat healthy food from all classes of food in the proportions outlined for you.

Generally, the food classes are:

1. **Vegetables,** which are subdivided into:

    a. **Non-starchy:** Examples include carrots, greens, peppers, tomatoes, and broccoli.

    b. **Starchy:** Examples are potatoes, corn, and green peas.

2. **Fruits:** Examples include melons, oranges, berries, bananas, apples, and grapes.

3. **Grains:** At least 50% of your daily grains should be whole grains, such as wheat, brown rice, oats, millet, cornmeal, barley, and quinoa. Examples are brown bread, popcorn, pasta, cereal, and tortillas.

4. **Protein:** Examples include:

    a. Lean meat (meat without fat)

    b. Skinless chicken or turkey

    c. Eggs

    d. Fish

    e. Dried beans

    f. Nuts and peanuts.

5. **Nonfat or low-fat dairy products:** Examples are yoghurt, milk, and cheese.

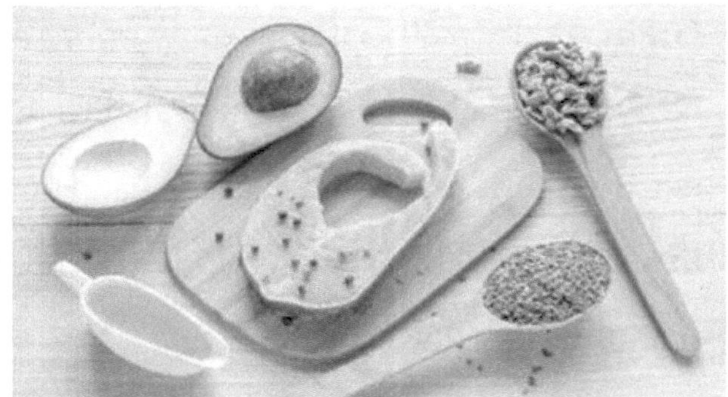

Recommended healthy fats such as from nuts, seeds, and olive oil.

Generally speaking, a healthy diet involves reducing calorie intake, replacing saturated fats with unsaturated fats, and consuming dietary fibers such as vegetables, whole grains, and fruits.

It also involves avoiding excessive alcohol intake, tobacco use, and added sugars.

Saturated fats are mainly found in animal foods, but they can also be found in some plant foods such as palm oil, palm kernel oil, and coconut. On the other hand, examples of unsaturated fats include avocados, olive oil, fish, soybean oil, and walnuts.

TYPE 1 DIABETES DIETS

People with Type 1 diabetes have an absolute insulin deficiency, which means their blood glucose levels can rise quickly. It is recommended that people with Type 1 diabetes consume foods with a low glycemic index, which measures how quickly a food raises blood glucose levels.

Foods with a low glycemic index raise blood glucose levels slowly, while those with a high glycemic index raise them quickly. For Type 1 diabetes, it is advisable to take insulin just before eating to ensure enough insulin in the body to absorb the glucose generated from the meal.

Specifically, the Mediterranean diet is recommended for people with Type 1 diabetes, which includes vegetables, fruits, fresh fish, and plant-based fats like olive oil and nuts. However, several foods should be avoided, such as those containing trans-fat, high-fat animal products, and anything labelled **hydrogenated.**

Simple carbohydrates, including processed or refined sugar, chips, cookies, and white bread, should also be avoided. Avoiding soft drinks, including regular and diet varieties, is also recommended.

TYPE 2 DIABETES DIETS

Vegetarian diets are often recommended for people with Type 2 diabetes. However, if you prefer not to eliminate meat, Mediterranean, and Paleo, keto diets are good alternatives as they contain less meat, fish, and dairy.

Regardless of which diet you choose, it should include a balanced mix of carbohydrates, proteins, and fats. Carbohydrates should mainly come from vegetables, while fats and proteins should come from plant-based sources.

To keep blood sugar levels stable, it's best to focus on complex carbohydrates with a low glycemic index and high protein content. This means consuming plenty of vegetables, fruits, oatmeal, lentils, and beans.

It's also essential to avoid foods with simple carbohydrates and processed foods high in sugar, such as white bread, white rice, pasta, soft drinks, and biscuits.

KETO DIETS FOR DIABETES

The keto or ketogenic diet is a high-fat, low-carbohydrate diet that is considered effective for weight loss and improving health. It has been found beneficial for people living with diabetes as it can reduce insulin resistance and improve sensitivity. However, it may increase the risk of hypoglycemia, especially for those with Type 1 diabetes.

The keto diet alters how your body stores and uses energy by encouraging the use of fat for energy generation instead of glucose or carbohydrates.

It is important to note that a keto diet should not be composed of only saturated fats but rather healthy monounsaturated and polyunsaturated fats found in vegetables and dairy products.

Therefore, your keto diet should consist of high levels of proteins, polyunsaturated and monounsaturated fats, including the following:

a. Avocado

b. Olives

c. Eggs

d. Natural cheeses

e. Lean meat

f. Sesame seeds

g. Unsweetened yoghurts.

Also avoid foods that contain a high level of saturated fats. Examples include the following:

a. starchy vegetable

b. Grains such as rice, pasta, and oatmeal

c. Soft drinks, whether regular or diet

d. Trans-fat-containing food such as margarine and deep fried foods.

e. Added sugars or sweeteners

You are strongly advised to consult your healthcare team before starting a keto diet. You should also monitor your blood sugar levels throughout the day to ensure they are within the expected target.

Therefore, you should NEVER embark on a keto diet if you are on insulin or oral diabetes medications without medical supervision, as it has life-threatening risks which includes severe hypoglycaemia and diabetic ketoacidosis.

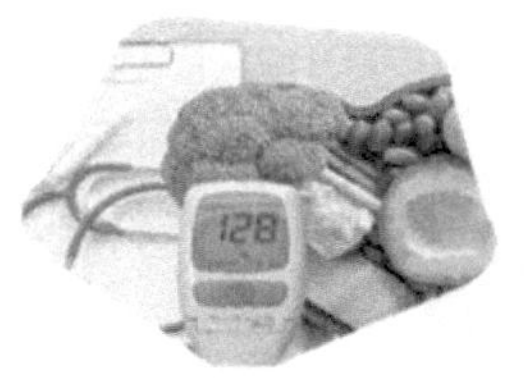

CHAPTER NINE

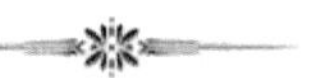

Diabetes and How It Can Affect Other Aspects of Your Health 1

"Even the darkest night will end and the sun will rise."

DIABETES AND YOUR MENTAL HEALTH.

Hearing about having diabetes for the first time can trigger what is known as diabetic distress. Diabetic distress refers to the mostly negative emotions you may experience when first diagnosed with diabetes.

Although this varies from person to person depending on their psychological makeup, you may feel sad, worried, guilty, or anxious about your diabetes. These feelings can occur from time to time.

Having these emotions about your diabetes is a normal, understandable, and natural reaction, as anyone newly diagnosed with a long-term medical condition like diabetes would feel the same.

Being aware of this can help you manage these feelings until you come to terms with your diabetes.

Furthermore, living with diabetes can be a burden, as it requires making various adjustments that can subsequently impact your life. These adjustments can take a toll on your mental health but know that you are not alone.

It is important to note that some of the root causes of diabetes distress, such as fear, anxiety, and negative emotions towards diabetes, stem from misconceptions about the condition, particularly concerning developing complications and managing the condition itself.

Your diabetes can lead to a mental health disorder, which in turn can negatively impact your ability to cope with and effectively take care of your diabetes - the most important aspect of managing the condition. This can create a vicious cycle.

Therefore, it is essential to pay attention to your emotions and discuss them with your healthcare providers, friends, family, or any other person or forum you feel comfortable with and can receive support from.

Your healthcare providers can provide information on coping and refer you to appropriate services when needed.

COPING WITH DIABETES DISTRESS

First, it's essential to know that having diabetes is common and nobody has a perfect experience with it. So, do not blame yourself or feel guilty for having it. Coping with diabetes distress involves the following steps:

a. Accepting and taking ownership of your diabetes. This will help you to be responsible for your care and find ways to manage your blood sugar level effectively.

b. Setting realistic goals for yourself regarding your blood glucose level control and blood test results. It is recommended to use words like 'high' or 'low' blood sugar rather than 'good' or 'bad' blood sugar to avoid feeling guilty or anxious.

c. Engaging in relaxation exercises such as meditation.

d. Expressing your emotions by talking to friends and family about how you feel and how they can support you. Connecting with others with the same condition can also be a helpful place to discuss diabetes and learn from their experiences.

e. Do not neglect your healthcare provider when you are experiencing diabetes distress. They can provide you with physical and emotional support, and together you can create a plan, including adjusting your routines to help you overcome or reduce your distress. Your healthcare provider will also inform you on how to cope and refer you to appropriate services when needed."

DIABETES BURNOUT

You may have put forth your best efforts to manage your diabetes, but sometimes, despite your hard work, you may not achieve the results you were hoping for, or you may develop a diabetes-related condition.

This can leave you feeling like all the measures, rules, and lifestyle changes you have followed were not worth it. You may feel discouraged, frustrated, and eventually, let down your guard and stop caring for yourself.

This is known as diabetes burnout, and it can lead to unhealthy habits such as neglecting to monitor your blood sugar level, consuming unhealthy diets, drinking, smoking, and missing appointments with healthcare providers.

If you experience diabetes burnout, taking the necessary steps to break the cycle is important. Remember what you're doing right and focus on what is working instead of paying attention to what is not working. Keep in mind that success stories are possible in the near future.

Most importantly, involve your diabetes care team and share your frustrations. They will be happy to help you and find a way forward.

DIABETES AND DEPRESSION

Sometimes, everyone feels low or sad, but these feelings usually do not last long, so they are a normal part of life. However, if you experience feelings of hopelessness, anxiety, and sadness for an extended period, especially two weeks or more, it could mean that you have developed depression.

Having diabetes puts you at risk of depression because it can cause feelings of being overwhelmed and exhausted, leading to long periods of feeling low, sad, or hopeless. There may also be a loss of interest in the things you previously enjoyed, a sense of worthlessness, poor sleep, or changes in appetite.

Talk to your healthcare provider if you have one or more of these symptoms for more than two weeks. Diabetes and depression share similar features, which can confuse one at arriving at the diagnosis. Tiredness, excessive sleep, and difficulty concentrating may occur with either condition or both, leading to uncertainty in diagnosis.

Having depression before diabetes can worsen your depression. Diabetes can exacerbate your depression through:

a. Worrying about controlling your blood sugar levels can be stressful.

b. Feelings of guilt, fear, and anxiety about diabetes.

c. Blaming yourself for poor blood sugar control.

Conversely, depression can negatively impact your diabetes through:

a. Feeling tired can make it difficult to exercise, which is essential for controlling blood sugar.

b. Self-neglect can lead to complications, such as not checking blood sugar levels, refusing to see a doctor, or not taking medications.

c. Not eating enough can put you at risk of hypoglycemia if you take insulin.

d. Overeating can cause your blood glucose level to rise.

e. Suicidal thoughts can make it challenging to take care of yourself.

Therefore, the relationship between diabetes and depression can become a vicious cycle. It's important to always talk to your healthcare professionals and seek help when needed. Do not try to hide your feelings or refuse help when offered.

COPING WITH DIABETES AND DEPRESSION

Discuss the available help you can access with your healthcare provider during your annual review or follow-up appointment. Managing your depression can involve both medical and non-medical approaches. Medical treatment includes taking antidepressants, which come in different classes.

Some work by enhancing serotonin levels in the brain to help improve your mood. Rest assured that safe antidepressants will be selected for you and will not negatively affect your diabetes.

Non-medical treatment options include exercising, which has a dual effect on depression and diabetes. You can also get support from friends and family members for both conditions.

Another option is Cognitive Behavioral Therapy (CBT), a form of psychotherapy involving structured discussions with a mental health counsellor over several sessions. CBT helps you understand negative thinking patterns that can negatively affect your emotions and behaviour and replace them with positive ones.

Your healthcare professional may start with non-medical treatment or combine medical and non-medical approaches for your depression management.

DIABETES SUPPORT GROUPS: BUILDING SOCIETY AND DISCOVERING HOPE

Diabetes support groups are community-based gatherings of people living with diabetes who interact together to share experiences, information, and provide emotional support for one another. The leaders of these groups can be healthcare professionals, volunteers, peer leaders, or simply be informal gatherings of people with diabetes.

Diabetes support groups can vary in forms or organizations, face-to-face meetings to online forums and social media groups.

Joining a diabetes support group is beneficial and has the following benefits:

1. **Emotional support:** living with diabetes can be lonely and distressing. Joining a support group can provide you a safe place to share your concerns.

2. **Advice:** support group can offer you practical advice on how to manage your diabetes in areas of medications, healthy lifestyle, and medication.

3. **Education:** this can be in forms of seminars, presentations, and reading materials with a view to give you the latest happening about diabetes management.

4. **Accountability:** Belonging to a support will help to be accountable and more responsible to your diabetes management.

HOW TO FIND A DIABETES SUPPORT GROUP

Finding a support group that suits you is not difficult as you can get by asking from your healthcare provider, searching online, looking for a local support group.

Diabetes support groups on Facebook include: Diabetes 101 for Beginners, Diabetes support group, Diabetes for young adults.

Other online diabetes support groups include: Diabetes Sisters, Diabetes Daily, Smart Patients, Beyond Type 2, etc.

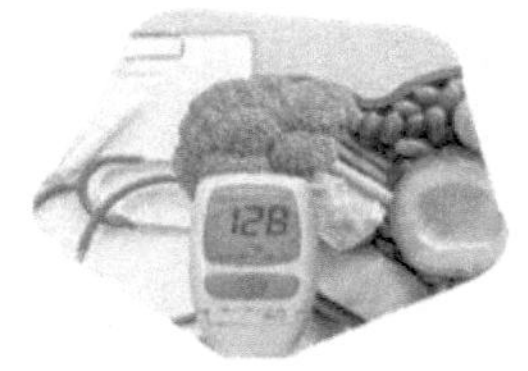

CHAPTER TEN

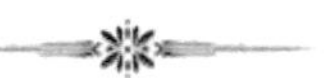

Diabetes and How It Can Affect Other Aspects of Your Health 2

DIABETES AND YOUR IMMUNITY

You have a higher chance of infection if you have diabetes because elevated blood sugar is known to depress immunity, thereby reducing your body's ability to control or combat harmful pathogens that enter your body.

Typically, your immune system consists of two major categories: innate immunity and adaptive immunity (also known as acquired immunity). Innate immunity is the one you are born with and includes barriers that protect your body against harmful pathogens, such as the skin, cough reflex, tears, mucus, and acid in the stomach. Innate immunity also includes chemical components such as interferon, interleukins-1, and complement.

Adaptive immunity is acquired over time through repeated exposure to pathogens. When a pathogen comes in contact with your body, your immune system develops a defense against that particular pathogen and keeps a memory of it. If that particular pathogen enters your body again, the already-formed immunity will quickly take care of it.

Adaptive immunity involves specialised blood cells and antibodies that attack harmful foreign agents and can remember and destroy them if they occur later.

In summary, innate immunity is the first line of defence, but if a harmful agent manages to bypass it, the adaptive immunity takes over.

HOW DOES DIABETES IMPACT YOUR IMMUNITY?

Patients with diabetes, especially if uncontrolled, have an increased risk of infections due to depressed immunity, as occasioned by the negative impacts of elevated blood sugar. The overall adverse effects of diabetes on the immune system occur through various mechanisms.

The competence of your skin, which is one of the constituents of the innate immunity, is significantly reduced, thereby allowing room for harmful organisms to enter the body.

Also, because of the nerve damage caused by diabetes and subsequent impairment of pain response, you may not notice any skin injury until the wound becomes infected.

As a person with diabetes, your skin's barrier immunity is compromised, making you more susceptible to skin and soft tissue infections.

If not properly managed, these infections can progress to osteomyelitis, a bone infection.

Additionally, poor blood flow to the infected area due to compromised blood vessels caused by diabetes can slow down wound healing and lead to further infections.

Elevated blood sugar levels also weaken your innate and adaptive immune systems, making you more prone to developing respiratory, skin and soft tissue, gastrointestinal, and genitourinary infections like urinary tract infections and vaginal candidiasis.

In summary, people with diabetes are more susceptible to infectious diseases due to the elevated sugar levels that compromise the body's barriers and reduce the production of defense chemicals needed to fight harmful bacteria and viruses.

Specific infections like Malignant otitis externa and Rhinocerebral Mucormycosis are unique to diabetes and can be life-threatening.

It's advisable to discuss with your healthcare provider the possibility of getting pneumococcal and influenza vaccines, which can reduce the risk of respiratory infections, hospitalisations, and death.

Finally, it's essential to avoid contact with anyone with chickenpox if you have not had it before or have not been vaccinated against it.

SICK DAY PLAN

Sick day plan simply means having a plan for your blood sugar control in case you fall ill. It helps you to manage your diabetes well and prevent complications.

Suppose you are down with a cold, flu, or diarrhoeal disease. In that case, the illness constitutes some sort of stress on your body, which in turn, responds by producing some chemicals that cause your blood sugar level to go up, making it challenging to keep your blood glucose controlled.

Having diabetes increases your risk of having a severe infection, but a sick day plan will help you navigate the period of the illness by reducing the risk of complications from the illness and allowing you to keep your blood sugar level within the normal range.

MANAGING YOUR BLOOD GLUCOSE LEVEL WHEN YOU ARE SICK

Getting your blood sugar level within the normal range is one of the best strategies to use to help your body overcome the illness. Elevated blood sugar during this time will further dampen your immunity which can in turn make your sickness more severe.

Therefore, you should develop a plan as to how to manage your diabetes and illness, should you fall sick. The plans should include the following:

a. How often you need to check your blood glucose level

b. What type of food to eat and drinks to take during the course of your illness

c. When do you need to call your doctor, especially if you have had three episodes of vomiting, diarrhoea, or fever greater than 101 degrees Fahrenheit or 38.3 degree Celcius in the past 24 hours?

d. How to adjust your insulin or OHAs

e. When to check for ketones

f. The kind of over-the-counter drugs you can take as some can elevate your blood sugar levels.

It is important that you write your down your plans and the medications you are currently taking so as to have something to fall back on.

It is will be good you watch out for symptoms of Diabetic Ketoacidosis (DKA) when you are sick, as your body may not produce enough insulin to catch up with increased demands of insulin which then puts you at risk of DKA.

Check for high ketones and high blood sugar more often. If you have high ketones in your urine but you have no sugar in your urine, it indicates that you are starved as what you are having is starvation ketosis. You should eat more and drink more fluid.

If you notice any symptoms of DKA, contact your doctor quickly.

DIABETES AND SURGERY

Surgery for someone having diabetes comes with a lot of challenges. Before and after surgery, you may require changes in your diabetes

regimen- whether insulin or oral medications- to ensure acceptable blood sugar level. This is to prevent complications such as slow healing and infections that can arise after the surgery.

Ensuring acceptable blood sugar levels when planning for surgery involves three stages:

Before Surgery.

While you are getting ready for surgery, you can do several things to ensure that your blood sugar level is well-controlled. These include:

i. Monitoring your blood sugar levels 2-4 times daily

ii. ii. Letting your healthcare provider know about your upcoming surgery. Your diabetes medications may need to be reviewed.

iii. If you are on Insulin, the dose may need to be adjusted a day before the surgery to prevent low blood sugar. Adhere to your doctor's instructions.

Your target blood sugar level should be between 80-130mg/dl before meals and less than 180mg/dl after meals.

During Surgery.

Surgery and anaesthesia can increase your blood sugar level. This is because surgery and anaesthesia increase the level of your stress hormones which in turn make your body less sensitive to insulin. This can result in increased blood sugar levels.

i.   If you have type 1 diabetes, you will require insulin during surgery.

ii.   ii. If you have type 2, you may still require insulin during surgery even if your diabetes is being managed with oral medication, exercise, and dietary modification.

After Surgery.

Depending on the type of surgery you did, you may not be able to eat or drink for some time. So, your dose or frequency of medications may need to be adjusted.

If you are staying in the hospital:

i.   You will be given a diabetic meal to ensure control of your blood sugar levels.

ii. Ii. If your blood sugar level is above 180mg/dl, you may be given insulin based on your healthcare provider's recommendation.

After you are discharged home:

i.   Ensure your blood sugar level is between 80-130mg/dl to promote healing and prevent infection.

ii. If your blood glucose level is above 200mg/dl, inform your doctor. Your medications may need to be reviewed.

iii. Do not skip your medication, whether insulin or oral medication, unless your doctor advises you to do so.

iv. Stick to an appropriate diet and drink sugar-free beverages to stay hydrated.

Note: If your glucometer is calibrated in mmol/L, you can convert it to mg/dl by multiplying the value you got in mmol/L by 18.

For example, if you check your blood sugar and it is 5mmol/L, then 5 x 18 is equal to 90.

Therefore, 5mmol/L is equivalent to 90mg/dl.

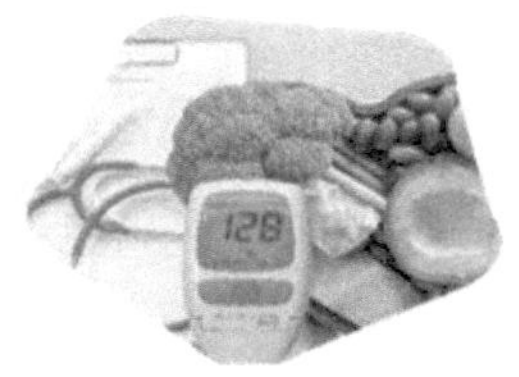

CHAPTER ELEVEN

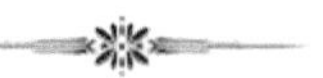

Diabetes in Pregnancy

DIABETES AND PREGNANCY

Diabetes can occur in pregnancy in two ways: pre-existing diabetes, which is when you have diabetes before getting pregnant, and gestational diabetes, which develops during pregnancy.

Pre-existing diabetes can be either type 1 or type 2, and discussing pregnancy plans with your healthcare provider is crucial. Poorly controlled blood glucose levels around the time of pregnancy can negatively affect both you and your baby, so it's essential to manage your condition carefully.

The effects of diabetes on your baby during pregnancy may include:

a. Birth defects

b. Restriction of your baby's growth

c. Too large birth weight

d. Preterm birth

e. Stillbirth

Getting pregnant with diabetes can also have an impact on you. You may risk developing pre-eclampsia, a potentially life-threatening condition in which your blood pressure is higher than normal and protein is found in your urine during pregnancy.

Additionally, giving birth to a baby that is too large (weighing greater than or equal to 10 pounds or 4.5 kg) may require a caesarean section.

GESTATIONAL DIABETES MELLITUS (GDM).

Gestational diabetes mellitus (GDM) is a type of diabetes that occurs for the first time during pregnancy in a woman who did not previously have diabetes.

It usually develops around 24 weeks of pregnancy and often does not have noticeable symptoms.

GDM is caused by pregnancy hormones produced by the placenta that oppose the action of insulin, leading to elevated blood sugar levels due to insulin resistance. It is important to note that GDM is not caused by a lack of insulin but by insulin resistance.

After delivery, GDM typically disappears, but having GDM does increase the risk of developing type 2 diabetes later in life. You may be monitored for persistent high blood sugar levels 6 to 12 weeks after delivery. Your doctor may recommend testing for GDM based on your medical history and risk factors.

Some risk factors increase the chances of developing gestational diabetes mellitus (GDM), including:

a. Being overweight or obese.

b. Having a family history of diabetes.

c. Being over 25 years of age.

d. Having prediabetes.

e. Having had GDM in a previous pregnancy.

f. Having polycystic ovarian syndrome (PCOS).

If you have GDM, there are potential risks to your baby, such as:

a. Being born larger than normal.

b. Being born earlier than expected.

c. Developing low blood sugar after birth.

However, these risks can be significantly reduced with proper management of blood sugar levels as soon as the diagnosis of GDM is made.

HOW IS GDM DIAGNOSED?

Gestational diabetes is usually diagnosed 24 to 28 weeks of pregnancy. Your doctor may decide to test you earlier if you have had it before or you have other things that put you at risk of having it.

Elevated blood sugar at the start of your pregnancy may mean that you have either type 1 or type 2 diabetes.

Oral glucose tolerance test (OGTT) is usually used to test for GDM.

TREATMENT OF GESTATIONAL DIABETES MELLITUS

Your doctor will individualise your treatment depending on:

a. Your age and overall health.

b. Your preference.

c. If you are able to tolerate specific treatment.

d. Severity of your GDM.

However, generally speaking, your treatment will aim at getting your blood glucose level controlled within the normal range and your doctor may commence you on the following:

a. Exercise

b. Healthy diet

c. Blood sugar monitoring

d. Insulin injections or metformin, as your case may require.

WHAT SHOULD YOU DO IF YOU ARE PLANNING TO BECOME PREGNANT?

You should see your doctor before getting pregnant so that appropriate plans can be mapped out for you, including preconception care.

You should generally do the following:

a. Ensure your HbA1c or blood glucose level is within normal range.

b. Take Folic Acid, a higher dose preferably, to reduce the risk of your baby developing a birth defect.

c. Maintain a healthy lifestyle.

d. Check your blood pressure and screen for other complications of diabetes.

Managing your diabetes will help you have a healthy pregnancy experience and a healthy baby.

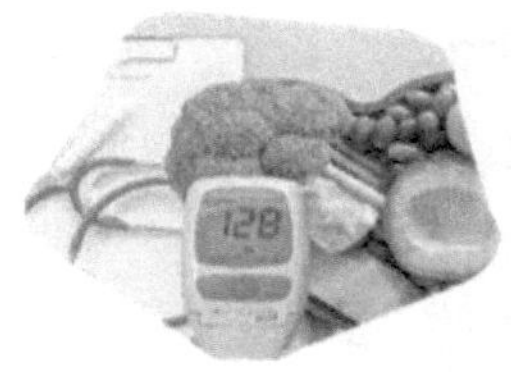

CHAPTER TWELVE

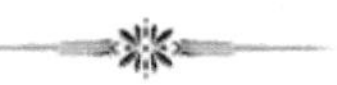

Prevention of Diabetes for Those at Risk

"Unlike viruses, bacteria, and infectious diseases, diabetes is not a disease. Either your genes or your lifestyle is to blame. Therefore, education rather than immunisation is needed to help prevent it. The norm is to educate people to eat well, recognise early warning signs, and not take anything for granted."- World Diabetes Day Awareness Slogans, 2022

PREVENTION OF DIABETES

Despite the pandemic level of diabetes, it's important to note that prediabetes and Type 2 diabetes can often be prevented.

You are at risk of developing diabetes if you are overweight or obese, have a parent or siblings that have diabetes, or have had prediabetes or gestational diabetes mellitus in the past. The longer you have diabetes, the more your risk of complications. Therefore, delaying it even for some years will enhance your life significantly.

You can delay or prevent diabetes by losing a fair amount of weight by eating food of low calories and being active most days of the week. Thus, staying lean and staying active is vital to preventing diabetes.

The following steps can help you reduce your chance of developing Type 2 diabetes

A. Have a weight-loss plan.

If you are overweight or obese, try to lose 5 to 10% of your weight within six months. For instance, if you weigh 200 pounds or 90kg, aim to lose 20 pounds or 9kg within six months, which is 10% of your weight.

To achieve your weight loss goal, it's recommended that you follow a healthy meal plan that includes low-fat, reduced-calorie meals and engage in physical activity. You should also adopt long-term changes that work for you.

Here are the four important steps to having a healthy weight-loss meal:

1. Eat food that has less saturated fat, trans fat, and added sugars.

2. Drink water instead of soda, fruit juice, and energy drinks.

3. Reduce your portion sizes of high-calorie, sugary, and fatty foods.

4. Replace unhealthy foods with healthier options.

The plate method is an effective way to control your portion sizes. Simply fill half of your plate with vegetables and fruits, one quarter with lean meat, and the other quarter with whole grains like brown rice or whole-wheat pasta.

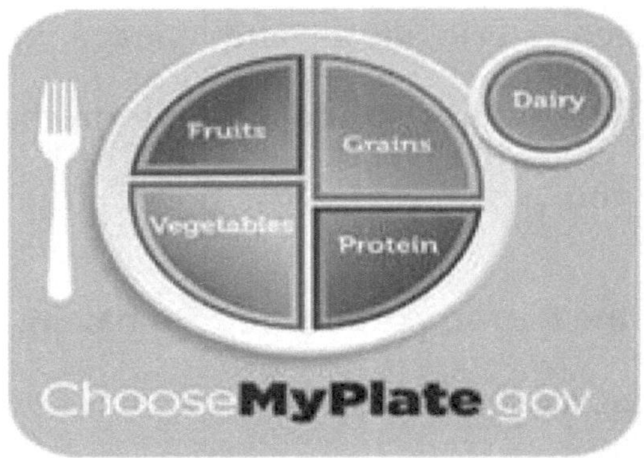

Source: U.S. Department of Agriculture.

You can also use familiar everyday objects or the size of your hand to measure the size of a portion. For instance:

i. 1 serving of meat or poultry is equivalent to the size of your palm or a deck of cards.

ii. A 13-ounce or 0.37kg serving of fish is about the size of a cheque book.

iii. Half a cup of pasta or cooked rice is a rounded handful or a tennis ball size

iv. Two tablespoons of peanut butter is a ping-pong ball.

Your meal plan should be comprised of different foods from each food class.

The diagram below helps you learn more about which foods to eat.

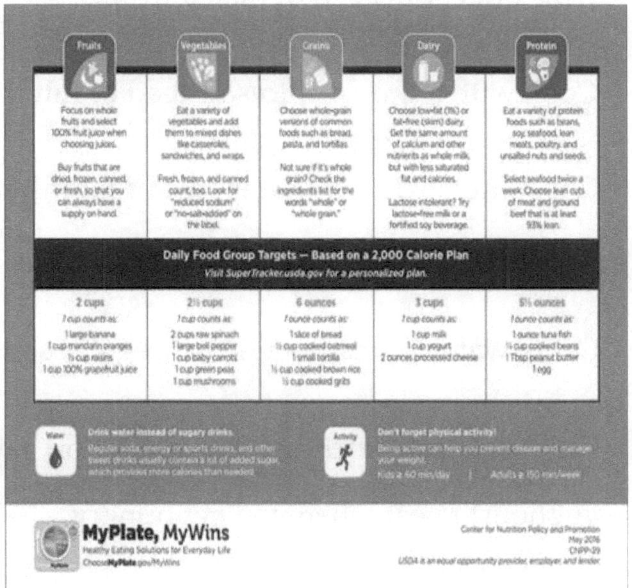

Source: U.S. Department of Agriculture

B Eating Tips for Weight Loss

i.   Get as close to your daily calorie goals as possible.

ii.   Eat meals on your smaller plates and keep your drinks in smaller glasses to make portions appear bigger.

iii.   Restrict your alcoholic beverages: Choose light wine or beer instead of mixed drinks.

iv.   Cook with a mix of spices instead of salt.

v.   Consume yoghourt that is free of fat instead of ice cream.

vi.   Drink water instead of juice or regular soda.

vii.   Pick a snack such as an apple or fat-free yoghourt to eat when you get hungry.

C. Increase Body Movement

Moving more each day helps you burn off more calories. This will help you attain your weight-loss plan and, at the same time, enable you to maintain it.

However, even if you cannot lose weight, staying active will help prevent or delay Type 2 diabetes.

It is recommended that you stay active for at least 30 minutes a day, five days in a week. A brisk walk is what is recommended for most people. But find out from your health care team the exercise that suits you.

Tips to help you get started and keep moving include:

i. **Dress to move:** This entails wearing shoes that fit well and enhance comfort, and dressing in clothing that allows for easy movement and keeps you dry and comfortable.

ii. **Start slowly:** Begin with 5-10 minutes of exercise you enjoy, gradually increasing the time to 30 minutes of moderate-intensity daily activity. Moderate-intensity activity improves heart and respiratory rates.

To gauge moderate-intensity activity, you should be able to speak but not sing while doing it.

iii. **Sit less in a day:** Stand up and move around every hour. While watching television, try to walk or dance around, or stretch.

iv. **Move your body more at work:** Take movement breaks more frequently at work. Use your lunch break to take a walk. Instead of sending an email to a colleague, deliver the message in person by walking to their desk.

Climb the stairs instead of using the elevator to your office. Consider setting an alarm to remind you to take movement breaks if you tend to forget.

v. **Count your number of steps per day:** Use a step counter or wearable electronic device, like a pedometer, to measure your steps. Aim for 7,000-10,000 steps per day.

vi. **Socialise:** Make your activities social by involving others, such as friends, family, or anyone who shares your goals. You can start a walking group with your neighbours, at your worship or work place. This will help you stay motivated and achieve your goals.

vii.   **Have fun:** Staying active does not have to be boring. Make your activities fun by playing music and dancing while doing household chores. Play sports with loved ones, such as children or grandchildren. Engage in swimming, walking, biking, jogging or any activity you enjoy.

viii.   **Keep your muscles strong:** Do weight lifting or use resistance bands two or more days a week to strengthen your muscles.

D. Do Not Smoke

Type 2 diabetes has been linked to the long list of health implications of smoking, as smokers have about a 50% chance of developing Type 2 diabetes. So, not starting to smoke or quitting smoking will help to prevent you from developing diabetes.

E. Reduce Your Alcohol Consumption

If you are already drinking alcohol, your goal should be to keep your consumption in the recommended moderate range, as anything higher than that could put you at an increased risk of developing diabetes. However, if you have not started drinking alcohol, you should not start.

Beyond The Individual Living With Diabetes.

Type 2 diabetes can largely be prevented by observing the principles of weight loss and control, increased exercise, moderate alcohol consumption, healthy eating, and avoiding smoking. However, it is crucial to recognise that the responsibility for lifestyle changes cannot solely fall on individuals with diabetes.

Therefore, families, friends, healthcare providers, school administrators, communities at all levels, the media, non-governmental organisations, governmental agencies, and the food industry must all work together to make healthy choices easier for people with or at risk of diabetes.

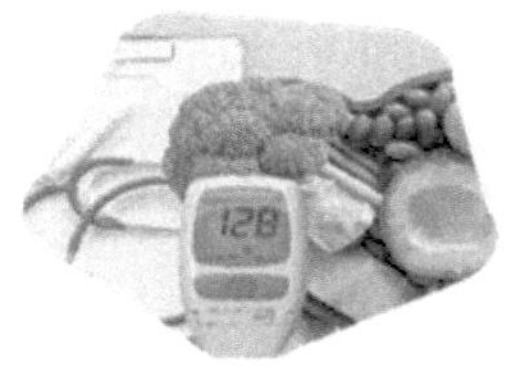

CHAPTER THIRTEEN

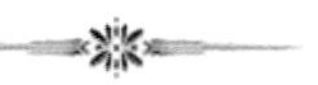

Debunking The Myths About Diabetes

"Diabetes is a complex but common disease. As its prevalence increases, it is essential to overturn myths as we find them."-MEDICAL NEWS TODAY

Diabetes has become a global pandemic. Unfortunately, many myths surrounding it have gained notoriety. This section aims to dispel any misconceptions about diabetes.

MYTH 1- EATING SUGAR CAUSES DIABETES

Although sugary diets can cause overweight and obesity which puts you at risk of developing diabetes, sugar does not directly cause diabetes.

MYTH 2- DIABETES IS NOT A SERIOUS CONDITION

Because diabetes is common, some think it is not a serious condition. This is incorrect because, apart from the fact that diabetes is not curable, many complications can arise from it.

MYTH 3- IT IS ONLY PEOPLE THAT HAVE OBESITY THAT DEVELOPS DIABETES

Obesity indeed puts one at risk of diabetes, but it also affects people of any body weight. About 11% of people who have diabetes do not have obesity. More so, Type 1 diabetes does not have any link with obesity.

MYTH 4- IT IS BETTER FOR PEOPLE WITH DIABETES TO COMPLETELY AVOID SUGAR

This is not true. You do not need to avoid sugar altogether. However, you do need to carefully consume healthy sugar even though you can use sweets as treats. ***"The key to sweets is to have a very small portion and save them for special occasions, so*** *you focus your meals on healthier foods."* - American Diabetes Association.

MYTH 5- YOU CAN CONTRACT DIABETES FROM SOMEONE ELSE

Diabetes is not a communicable or infectious disease such as cold or flu. Therefore, you cannot contract it from someone else.

MYTH 6- IF YOU START USING INSULIN TO CONTROL YOUR DIABETES, IT MEANS YOU HAVE FAILED

This is not true. Using insulin to control your blood sugar level is not a bad thing. Initially, dietary management, oral medications, and exercise can control your blood sugar level.

However, Type 2 diabetes can be progressive. Along the line, your body may start producing less and less insulin, and at this point, oral medications will no longer suffice to achieve target control.

MYTH 7- PEOPLE WITH DIABETES NEED SPECIAL FOOD

No. You do not need to eat special because you have diabetes.

Besides being more expensive, foods that are termed "diabetes-friendly" can still elevate your blood sugar level.

Your healthy meal plan is the same for everyone; many dietary plans can help you. Ensure your diet includes non-starchy vegetables, whole grains, and limited added sugars. You should also pay attention to unsaturated fatty foods instead of saturated ones.

MYTH 8- YOU SHOULD NOT DRIVE IF YOU HAVE DIABETES

This is not the case. People with diabetes can drive. However, if you have visual problems, see your healthcare provider for assessment.

MYTH 9- THERE ARE NATURAL PRODUCTS THAT CAN CURE DIABETES

Currently, there is no known cure for diabetes, and any narrative that a herbal product can cure diabetes is untrue. Herbal or natural products, vitamins and supplements can even interact with your diabetes medications, whether oral or insulin, increasing your risk of hypoglycaemia.

MYTH 10- OBESITY ALWAYS CAUSES DIABETES

While it is true that obesity increases your risk of developing diabetes, it does not absolutely cause diabetes.

MYTH 11- SINCE NO ONE IN the FAMILY HAS DIABETES, I CAN NOT HAVE IT

You are at increased risk of developing diabetes if any of your first-degree relatives have it. However, lots of people with diabetes do not have a family history of diabetes.

MYTH 12- ONCE MY BLOOD SUGAR IS WITHIN TARGET LIMITS; I CAN STOP TAKING MEDICATIONS

Diabetes, as of now, does not have any cure. If you stop taking medications, your blood sugar can become dangerously high. So, if your blood sugar level is under control, continue taking your medications as advised by your health care provider.

MYTH 13- SINCE ANTS DO NOT GATHER AROUND MY URINE, I DO NOT HAVE DIABETES

This is a false claim. The only way to know you do not have diabetes is to do a blood sugar test.

****
158

Thank you for reading this book. I will love to hear from you. Kindly send your feedback to festust20@gmail.com or leave me a review at your favourite bookstore. Thanks

****